BEND OVER

Medical Stories You Won't Forget

John Bankhead
Vincent Frattaruolo

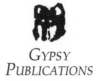

GYPSY
PUBLICATIONS

Published in 2019, by Gypsy Publications
Troy, OH 45373, U.S.A.
www.GypsyPublications.com

First Edition

These stories are based on the authors' best recollection of events. While the stories included in this book are non-fiction and based on actual events, the names, identifying characteristics, and locations appearing in this work have been changed to protect the respective individual's privacy.

The opinions expressed in this book are those of the authors and are not necessarily those of the publisher.

Bankhead, John
Frattaruolo, Vincent
Bend Over: Medical Stories You Won't Forget
by John Bankhead & Vincent Frattaruolo

ISBN 978-1-938768-90-3 (paperback)

DEDICATION

This book is dedicated to all of the hardworking nurses who toil every day trying to render good care despite the obstacles placed in their path by management. Twelve hour shifts in hospitals, driving your own car on your own gas doing home health visits, Low pay, old equipment, no lunch, no breaks, not allowed to sit down, get your own coverage so you can go to the bathroom, and a host of other things I don't have room to mention. Abused by arrogant Physicians, demanding patients and families, threatened by management, and assaulted by demented patients every day.

Today nurses graduate from one of the myriad of nursing schools, work a year or two, and go back to jobs they had before nursing. They won't work in a profession who's motto is "nurses eat their young."

Bless each and every one of them.

Table of Contents

PROLOGUE

Lots of things come to mind reflecting on my career in nursing, almost all of them bad. The other side of things, the good, were the dedicated people I worked with every day in the hospital hallways. These were the people who made medicine live and breathe every day, the ones who suffered with the patients through some of the worst experiences in their lives. The doctors were occasional visitors who came and went, but the nurses made it happen day in and day out. They received no monetary compensation worthy of their sacrifice, no thanks, no recognition for their good work, nothing, yet they showed up every day.

Like soldiers, they were in a battle, and some were injured, and disabled, yet they received no pension, no free medical care, and were cast out on the street to fend for themselves. There was no justice for any of them, they were attacked from all sides. The patients who scratched them, bit them, struck them, kicked them, cursed at them, yet they still rendered care to those who abused them daily. The arrogant doctors who couldn't function without them, belittled their knowledge, refused them common courtesy, and refused to even look at them when they passed in the hallway. Hospital administrators who made the nurses stand in the hallway all day, and then increased the shifts to 12 hours so they had to stand for 4 hours longer. The supervisors who refused to pay aides so the nurses had to administer meds late because they were changing beds until lunch, which they never got to eat. To go to the bathroom when working, meant you had to provide your own coverage using another nurse who was just as overworked as you. Try to cover an additional six patients at either ends of a long hall, with 3 of your own lights on. Work a year under these conditions an attend a review where they offer you a 10 cent raise for a years dedicated work. Enjoy working when you find every new hire is making more money then you and you have been there for five years and are told "if you don't like it, go somewhere else." You do go somewhere else, and it's the same shit on a different day only this time you get a 25 cent offer, and the new hires are still making more than you.

Switch to home health and you use your own car without compensation for it. They say "take it off on your taxes" like they know how taxes work, and they don't. Like working in the ghetto where you have to keep your feet moving so the roaches don't run up your legs. The entire experience makes you very good at what you do, but you are so fed up with it all that the money is never worth it, and you look for something else to do. Hopefully something where you will be appreciated, even a little bit, would be nice.

WHY DID I BECOME A NURSE

By John Bankhead RN,BSN (retired)

Why did I choose to become a nurse? The story started when I took a winter vacation in Clearwater Florida. At the time, I was working for AVIS Rent A Car at Philadelphia International airport. I was Damage Control Manager for Philadelphia Zone. My position gave me a company car which allowed me to use a company vehicle while on vacation. After several moves between hotels, I wound up in a motel on Clearwater Beach directly across from a refreshment stand on the beach, it was wonderful. We spent a week there, and eventually had to go back to the airport and turn in my car to catch a flight home to Philadelphia. While on the plane I thought how nice it was in Clearwater, and how lucky people were to live there all the time. It was then that I had a though that if other people could find a way to live there, why couldn't I? After returning home, I spent a lot of time thinking about making a move to Clearwater possible.

I decided to try to move inside AVIS Rent A Car and contacted the manager at Tampa Airport about a move. He assured me that there was no chance of that happening, and I was not the first person in the country to get that idea. I then thought of working for a car dealership, but could se no longevity or money in that job, so I crossed that one off. I had significant medical training from my time as a paramedic in the Philadelphia Fire Dept. so I began to ask around about my chances at nursing school. Unfortunately, nursing school required college, and I had flunked out of college when I was eighteen.

I decided after talking to a nurse that I would give college a try again. I enrolled in community College and took the placement tests. I scored well, so I was allowed to take any college courses I wished without remedial work. I got a copy of the requirements for admission into the nursing program, and decided to start with those classes first. Surprisingly, I did very well and decided that I would double up on classes to finish the program faster. Then I found out that there were pre summer classes, summer classes, and post summer classes, so I took all those too. As I ticked off the required classes I became more confident about my ability to be successful at nursing.

I applied to several nursing schools in the City and waited for my acceptance letters to come in. The first one I received was from Episcopal Hospital School of Nursing. I met with the faculty and agreed to enroll in the next class. At the same time, I saw a notice that a university was accepting students who had completed all prerequisite courses, and was holding interviews near my home, so I went with my transcript to check it out. The university had rented a space for several days to interview prospective students. I took my paperwork and sat for the interview, not realizing at the time it was a very expensive Ivy League School. I talked with the recruiter (who was actually an instructor in the school who I would have later in my studies) who looked over my transcript and to my astonishment committed to enrolling me in their next class, despite being short on the credits they required for admission. She listed what I needed to fill out my transcript and most of those were electives which I had not taken due to concentrating on core requirements. I was in trouble with two subjects, Food and Nutrition Science, and a year of basic College Biology. I was given one year to complete the 16 credit hours I was short, while attending nursing classes at Thomas Jefferson University with a full load of credits. Jefferson required 60 credit hours for admission, so I was admitted provisionally until I could fulfill all of the requirements. I was required to see a counselor as part of my provisional status, and when I arrived, he had my college transcripts and was astonished at the requirements I had to fulfil. He told me that I would have to look into CLEP to get the credits while attending Jefferson classes. I had no idea what CLEP (college level examinations) was so I inquired. I found out that I could get credit for a course by paying the course fee, and sitting for the final exam without taking the classes. I decided to try, so I took an advanced psych course. I aced the test and got 3 credit hours added to my transcript. I found a course which replaced the year of Biology, so I enrolled and aced that test and scratched that one off. I found a Food and Nutrition Science course at a local junior college, and ticked another off, then I went nuts. I enrolled in every CLEP course they had which even came close to a medical discipline, and even took business law and aced that too, I passes all of them and knocked off all the Jefferson electives I needed too. The last CLEP course I took was business, but I missed it by two questions, so I decided to stop taking CLEP courses. My secret for passing them was to buy the course book and read the end of chapter summaries and tests before the exams, and it worked.

When the year of my provisional admittance passed, I had completed every one of the 16 credit hours I needed, and all of the elective credits required for my Jefferson degree. My provisional status was cancelled, and I proceeded on as a full status student in the nursing program. 50% of the coursework at Jefferson was writing, reports, case studies, research, scientific papers, etc. You needed to score well on these reports to pass each subject, errors on a paper were fatal. A student received a 10 point deduction for even a misplaced comma, and a misspelling was a fatal flaw that could kill your mark. I hired a typist to do my papers. I would do all the work, and submit the hand written 20 pages (all reports must be at least 20 typewritten pages in length) to the typist, who would give a rough draft back to me. I would review it and hand it back with corrections, the typist would repeat the process one more time, and then print and bind the report to be turned in, I always got between 98 and 100.

During the classes, students seldom raised issues about the subject matter taught, especially if the instructor held strong opinions on the subject. Most of the students had no prior medical training, so, they accepted everything said as fact, including the instructor's personal opinions on subjects.

Well, that was not going to get past me, especially if I had a differing opinion. I thought that a university setting was the place for discussion, and using the Socratic method was acceptable, horse shit. An instructor took issue with me over a discussion in class, and gave me a 60 on my 20 page report. She could find no errors of any kind, so she said that she didn't feel that the subject matter was exactly what she expected. I was called to her office for a meeting the outcome is mentioned in one of the stories. The issue was resolved to my benefit, and I moved on to graduate as a bachelor of science in nursing. This gave me a license to practice nursing as a Graduate Nurse, until the first licensure exam. It also allowed me to fulfill my aspiration of moving to Clearwater Florida as a nurse, which took me 5 years from start to finish. So there you have it, I became a nurse so that I could get a job in my new locale, I did not hear a "calling" I was not "destined to help people" or "preordained" I wanted to earn money doing what I had experience doing which was what I was trained to do, I didn't have to like it, and I didn't.

WHY DID I BECOME A NURSE
By Vincent Frattaruolo RN, BSN, MS

The reason I became a nurse was economics, which is why most people go into nursing. I admit there are a few people like my wife who dreamed of being nurses from childhood, but most people do not. In childhood, people have other aspirations than nursing. Suctioning a trachea, changing dirty dressings or cleaning an incontinent patient is not glamorous. What you do goes largely unappreciated.

For me, the road to nursing begins when I was in the Air Force. My commanding officer had a friend who was a college counselor. One day when we were in town together, we ran into his friend. He said "Vince is leaving the Air Force what do you think he should do"? She responded "go into nursing." She said there were no men in her college's nursing program and no women in the engineering program. She stated "if we had a male in the nursing program or a woman in the engineering program, they would have no problem finding a job."

After leaving the Air Force, I returned to Florida and worked at a department store selling fine jewelry. I enjoyed being a jewelry salesman, but I did not want to do it for the rest of my life, so applied to law school. I was accepted to the University of Georgia School Of Law and the University Of Ohio School Of Law. I was not too thrilled about going to law school because I heard there was an overabundance of lawyers. One day while having dinner at a local restaurant I overheard a conversation two young women at the next table were having. Both women were secretaries married to lawyers. Both women said they were making more money than their husbands. That conversation clinched it for me; I was not going to law school. Meanwhile everyday there were dozens of ads in the newspaper for nurses, but I never saw an ad for a lawyer. I remembered what the college counselor said, so I began investigating nursing.

When I told my mother, I was thinking of becoming a nurse she suggested I talk to her friend Kathy who was an R.N. Kathy told me there was a nursing shortage (from 1978 to 2008 the U.S experienced a nursing shortage). She suggested that I work as a nurse's aide first to see if I like nursing. I had two older customers who were retired nurses. Both women told me that they worked throughout the Great Depression. I thought in retail, I am subject to the whims of the economy. If there is a recession and jewelry sales drop, I could easily lose my job. Nursing would provide me with economic stability. Next, I went to the local hospital and spoke to the nurse who was in charge of education. She explained the salary ranges for nurses and told me about the various nursing programs in the area.

After completing my nurse's aide course, I left the department store. I have been working in nursing ever since (thirty-eight years). I spent three years working as an aide, three years as a L.P.N. and thirty-two years as a R.N. While in nursing I was never unemployed. I was able to grow intellectually. The hospital paid for my bachelor's degree in nursing and my M.A. in library science. As an R.N., my salary provided me a comfortable life. I was able to purchase a new car every four years, buy a condo, and pay off a thirty year mortgage in fifteen years, travel, date, put money away for retirement and after I got married my wife did not have to work. Interesting enough one of the R.N.s I work with is a former lawyer.

BEING A HOME HEALTH RN
Did you report this to the visiting nurse?

When I transferred from working on the floor of a hospital, I moved to home health nursing. Home health nursing requires the nurse to travel from house to house administering care prescribed in advance by a physician. There are many reasons for prescribing home healthcare, and almost all of them are abused in one way or another. In many cases the doctor is doing a favor for a patient, the patient's family, church, friends of his, or he just doesn't want to understand the rules connected with home health care. Additional abuses come in the form of the home health agency, or home health nurse, continuing a patient on home healthcare when it is absolutely no longer needed. This story is about an abuse of this type that went wrong.

A home health nurse is assigned a certain amount of patients to see every day, the appointments for those patients are usually made the night before by telephone. Each patient that you see has been admitted to home healthcare by a registered nurse. This means you went to their home and interviewed them to determine their need for services, which are provided by the agency you work for. The services can be a registered nurse, a home health aide, supplies, physical therapy, occupational therapy, social worker and many other services. The registered nurse is the gatekeeper for all services provided in the home. The doctor has specified most of the services in his discharge orders. Once the services have been completed and the patient is functioning independently, one by one the services can be discontinued, until all of the agency personnel are out of the home for good.

A nurse going on vacation requested that I handle some of his caseload while he was away. He was dividing the caseload up against three nurses each to cover a portion of his cases. At the time I was given three of his patients to add to mine, and agreed to see them in his place. The next day I went to see the first of his patients which was located on the second floor of a condo complex with no elevator. This means that you hump your bag and pertinent equipment up to the second floor and walk down to the unit at the other end of the building. The unit is never near the stairs and the stairs are never near where your car is parked. When I entered his condominium, I greeted the patient, and I asked him several questions, one of which was why he was being seen every day. With that he produced a scar on his chest on the left side which was thoroughly healed. He informed me that the nurse was seeing him because he had had a pacemaker installed. After reviewing his chart to verify the information I was given, I told him that the pacemaker site was completely healed and there was really no need for me or anyone else to visit him every day. He said he would be sorry to see the nurses go, because the nurse sat down every day for about an hour and they just talked, no care was being given. Without further ado I discharged the patient from home health services and proceeded to the next case.

I found out later that the Home Health Agency cancelled the discharge, and reassigned the patient to another RN to illegally milk the insurance company and Medicare. This was common practice with every patient I discharged from home health. Some were milked for a week or so, and others were milked for several months, whatever they could get away with. The RN's were complicit in the scheme because they got paid for doing nothing but driving around in their cars. They kept a few RN's like me around to do the grunt work like admitting them to services, dumping the hard cases on, going into "bad" neighborhoods, and visiting "pain in the ass patients."

The next case was located in a condominium just around the corner from the first, and this time it was on the first floor which made it quite easy. I was admitted to the home by a man in his early 70s who was limping around with a bandage on his foot. Again, I asked the gentleman why he was being seen, and he showed me a healed scar on his body from a minor surgery. He wasn't at all concerned about the minor surgery, he was more concerned about the pain in his foot, so I agreed to examine it. He informed me that several days prior he had been out walking and had suddenly experienced a very sharp pain in his right foot. He reported that when he limped home, he pulled off his shoe and sock, and found an open sore on his foot. The sore was circular a little over a half inch in diameter, located on the outside of his foot near the sole of the foot. I asked the patient "did you report this to the visiting nurse", and he said he had, as the nurse visited him shortly after he returned from the walk. The nurse had talked to his physician about it that very day. I reviewed the chart in the house and found that the visiting nurse I was covering for, had reported the problem as a venous stasis ulcer, and had received treatment orders from the physician for that problem. Immediately I knew there was a problem with this wound that was not being addressed. The wound was not a venous stasis ulcer, it was an arterial ulcer, which means the blood supply to that area of the foot has been compromised. When this happens, you have four hours to rectify the problem and reestablish the blood supply to the affected area. I informed the patient that I didn't like the way the foot looked, as it was bluish purple in the area of the ulcer. I decided immediately I was going to call his nurse as soon as I left the home. When I got outside, I called his nurse on the phone told him about the misdiagnosis that he had made on the foot, and informed him that this problem needed his immediate attention. I had to leave a message on the phone as he did not answer the phone. I wanted to give the nurse the opportunity to correct his problem on the spot, because he had made several very serious mistakes in this case. Firstly, instead of sending the patient directly to the doctor's office or the hospital, he had diagnosed the problem himself, and gave the doctor the diagnosis over the telephone, which was wrong. Secondly, since nurses are not allowed to diagnose problems, he was practicing medicine without a license, which is illegal. Since the patient had had the problem for several days, essentially the damage was done because the problem was not handled immediately when it was found. I went out on a limb calling the nurse on the phone and giving him an opportunity to straighten out the mess and make things right. First thing the next morning, I found out that I had indeed made a mistake in trusting the nurse to do the right thing. I was called into the boss' office and dressed down for getting the patient upset. After I had informed the patient that I did not like the look of his foot, he started making calls about it. I was further informed by the supervisor that the nurse who had been visiting the patient for over a month knew much more about the patient's condition than I could ever know with one visit. I was further informed that because of this incident the other visiting nurse had filed a complaint against me with the agency. The supervisor further informed me that I would be put on probation from this point forward, and any incidents similar to this would result in my dismissal. I couldn't understand what had happened, other than the fact that the other visiting nurse was lying to the supervisor about everything. I was not allowed to rebut the argument with my own version of the events. The decisions had all been made before I was called to the office.

I went about my work seeing my patients while making plans to revisit this case in a week or two after receiving my tongue lashing. The time passed without incident, and I was retained on probation until one day several weeks later, I had an opportunity to go into the file room and pull the chart on the patient I had seen that day. I sat down at a table in the file room and read the chart including all the notes written after I had made my entry two weeks before. What I read filled me with disgust, and caused me to lose a lot of faith in the nurses I was working with. This nurse ignored the arterial problem on his patient for two more days, whereupon he made a phone call to the physician and reported that there was a change in the patient's status and that he now had an arterial ulcer and needed to be seen. The doctor told the nurse to call 911 and have the patient taken immediately to the hospital emergency room where he would meet him. The patient was admitted to the hospital, and various studies were performed. A section of his foot was considerably discolored because it'd been without blood for an extended period of time. I picked up the chart walked into the supervisor's office and laid it on her desk. I went to tell her that my diagnosis on the patient was correct and that the other nurse had lied about the patient's condition which ultimately resulted in a partial foot amputation. The supervisor taken aback, refused to read the chart, and essentially forced me out of her office. I left, leaving the chart behind, resolving that I would not work for her going forward. While in the office I further stated that she needed to give me an apology for doubting my competence. The next day I was informed that I was being removed from probation, we were going to forget the whole thing, but I wasn't going to forget the whole thing. I left on two weeks vacation that weekend, and refused to go back to the job. When I called to give my two weeks notice, I was connected to the supervisor who informed me that I was to return from vacation and work an additional two weeks before I could leave. Since I was just starting the two week vacation and had already secured another job at a Chevrolet dealership I refused. She stated that she would put a do not hire on me if I refused to follow her orders. We went round and round over it for several minutes, and I told her to do whatever she wanted to do and hung up on her. She placed a do not hire on me with the entire hospital network. I was later able to circumvent the do not hire by working for agencies and getting assignments to work all over the system she banned me from.

HOLY CRAP THEY'RE EVERYWHERE

I knew where the money for that job had gone!

At this point you are probably wondering how an RN got a job at a big Chevrolet dealership. I had previously held a position with AVIS RENT A CAR as Damage Control Manager for Philadelphia Zone. I had all the necessary Pennsylvania State Licenses for that position. The personnel department at the dealership accepted my qualifications and assigned me a team of autobody men to repair the cars that I wrote estimates on. I secured the job outside nursing while I was on vacation from the home health position.

Briefly moving ahead to my job at the Chevrolet dealership, I found I had walked into a hornet's nest of disgruntled employees. I had taken the place of a service advisor who had walked out of the job in the middle of the week before. It seemed that the manager who had hired me was hated by the employees. I was informed almost immediately, by the others that worked in this department, that the manager was at the root of all the problems. Since I had only worked there a couple days, I resolved not to get involved and just do my job. This dealership functioned on a team system, with one service advisor having a group of five technicians that he was to write and assign the work to. Each autobody man had a three car bay that was filled with the jobs he was working on until they were completed, then a new job would be assigned. I was to greet customers as they came in to have damage repaired, write the job, and drive it over to my team in the shop, and assign it to one of my autobody men. I knew every job that was assigned because I had written the ticket on every job. I would visit the body repair area every few hours to check progress on my jobs, and try to keep things moving along. Problems were addressed, and finished jobs were inspected before the customer was called.

There were three teams working in this shop, with each damage writer doing the same thing, with the same size team. The manager of the department did not have much to do except get himself into trouble because the system worked pretty well. I was there a little over a week when I noticed something odd, a car was pulled into one of my work areas that I didn't write a ticket on. I asked the technician where that car had come from, and he told me that the body shop manager had given it to him, and that it was a rush job, so he let my cars sit and worked on this one. I asked him to see the ticket (appraisal) on the job that the body shop manager had written, and he responded that he did not have one. Since there was no ticket on the job there was no way for the dealership to get paid for all the parts, labor, and material used on the job, because they were all listed on the ticket. I went over to the body shop manager's office and asked him for the ticket on the car he had assigned to my crew. He became somewhat irate, and told me "don't worry about it, I'm taking care of it." I told the manager that one of my crew was working on that car, and I wanted my crew credited for all the work performed on that vehicle because the tickets I had written were not being worked on. The manager again told me "I said don't worry about it." I smelled a rat right away, and assumed that my technician was punched in on one of my jobs and was instead working on the job for the body shop manager. This meant that all the labor, parts, and materials was billed out against one of my legitimate jobs while this "rush" job was done by the dealership for free. The "rush" job was a cash job and the body shop manager was collecting the cash.

Days later I went to the cashier Vanessa with all the information on the car that was the "rush" job. I had copied down the ID number, tag no. vehicle make, model and color on the job and handed her the information. I asked her if the ticket on that job was processed through her, and she said that she couldn't find anything on the job, which had left the dealership two days before. I knew where the money for that job had gone, right into the pocket of the body shop manager.

Two days later another car appeared in my area, and again there was no ticket on the job. I again went to the body shop managers office and asked for the ticket on the job to which he answered again "don't worry about it." At this point I knew that I was in the middle of a series of illegal transactions undermining the entire body shop operation. At lunch I discussed with the other estimators, and they informed me that the same thing was going on in their teams all the time. I had a problem, being a part of a scheme where large sums of money were being taken out of the business. I also had a problem that everyone knew about it and played along because they could not afford to get another job somewhere else. I also found out that the fellow I replaced had discovered the scheme and quit because of it. I had definite concerns that should everyone be questioned by the authorities, my nursing license could be involved if I faced charges as an accessory. I quit the job and went back to cardiac nursing, getting a job in one day.

I found out later from an employee I worked with, that the manager was found out, someone ratted him out and he was fired. I assumed it was one of the other appraisers who knew what was going on.

LIE CHEAT STEAL
That's not how I work

Transferring from working on a hospital floor to home health is a different experience. You report to an office usually located in a hospital owned medical office building, or a leased office building. This building, wherever it's located contains a large medical file room, a meeting room, and some offices for the supervisors who each has a cadre of nurses who do the visiting of the patients, and actually make the money for the agency. Smart agencies keep the non- money-making employees to a minimum. These privately run outfits are very efficient and use a lot of well trained agency nurses to staff their daily visits. They have minimal full time visiting nursing staff which do all the patients that are grouped a short distance from one another, and can be seen and dealt with quickly. The agency nurses usually visit the problem cases and those out in the sticks.

Now we get to the hospital based, home health departments. These departments are usually top heavy with supervisors, poorly managed, and take every opportunity to milk the system for everything it is worth. They do this, to make a profit because they are inefficient and need to pay lots of staff that see no patients unless they can make a quick buck on one on their way into work, something easy to do. There are also physicians who "make deals" with the hospital based home health departments promising to give them work if they will "take care" of friends or family that really shouldn't be on home health. These are two of those stories;

The hospital based unit I was working for at the time, had a home health RN who was a semi-professional swimmer. Every so often she would have to fly to an event to compete nationally, so nurses would have to cover her patients while she was away. She was an agency favorite, which meant that she was well connected in the office and received all of the do-nothing cherry-picked work. Somehow, I received one of her cases to visit along with my regular case load. Of course, that was a big mistake on the part of the office, assigning her case to me. I was supposed to know that her patients should be sat on until she returned and handed back with no changes whatsoever, but that's not how I work.

I made my first visit to the patient in question which was located two city blocks from the other nurse's house. In the house were two people, a husband and his wife. The wife was on full home health, with full time hospital aids, and an RN daily, and I was to be the RN for the week. When I entered the house, I reviewed the chart and saw that the wife received 1 unit of insulin with every visit. I did the vital signs and administered the one unit of insulin as directed by the doctor's orders. The wife asked me to fill her husband's med minder, and "would I please give him his daily medications with a glass of water." He was not my patient, and there was no reference to him at all in the chart on the table. The wife told me that the swimmer did this for her when she came daily, so I did her a favor and gave the meds.

This scenario went on uninterrupted until the third day when I smelled a rat, who the hell gets 1 unit of insulin and no finger sticks to check blood sugar??? I suspected that this patient was being used to bilk Medicare by the office. I was in the kitchen charting when the home health aide came in the back door with two grocery bags and put them on the table near me. She opened the freezer door and started unloading ice cream sandwiches, Dixie cups, and ice cream popsicles into the freezer. I immediately asked her what she thought she was doing with all that ice cream. Her face turned red and she called the wife into the kitchen. They both looked like they had been caught with their hand in the till. I picked up the phone and called the physician. I got the doctor on the phone and related the discovery to him, and asked why she had one unit of insulin ordered which did nothing at all. I further related that the refrigerator was full of ice cream which both her and her husband must be eating. The doctor asked me where the swimmer was, and I told him she was out of the state for a week. He said that he would call to the office and take care of it immediately. When I got back to the office, I found that the case had been reassigned to another nurse to cover. I also heard that the only reason anyone went to the house was to fill the husband's meds, and make sure he took them daily, as he was senile which I saw when I was in the house. The joke was that he was never the patient, ever, yet we were giving insulin 1 unit to his wife so he could get the free service from the RN and this event was a regular thing with this job, I was the exception. Time after time I would discharge a patient only to have the agency send out another nurse to readmit them to home health. There is not much need for honest people in hospital based home health.

MOM, BEND OVER
The spot on her buttocks had been there for years

In this visit, the home health case was in a very large complex of buildings on the first floor at the end of the row. Inside were an aged mother and her retired son who had a massive problem himself, but the son was not the patient. The patient was the mother, and when I did my initial visit, I had a problem with why I was sent out to see them. The mother had a spot on her behind that the son said she had been suffering with for years. I examined the mother and there was a small area less than a dime on her buttock cheek. It looked like a partially healed area that really presented no danger of infection. It was regular skin colored area that seemed to be kept from closing completely by wet diapers the mother wore. Along with my visit was a home health aide who bathed the mother every other day. I decided that I would find a way to get this spot to close or die trying.

When I went back to the office, I went into the chart room and looked up the past treatments given to the mother by the staff. I found volumes of charts going back 10 years or more where the mother was a patient of home health each winter. The story in the chart went as follows;

The mother lived with the son who was present in the apartment, and both were snow birds (winter only residents) in Florida. They lived in a condo unit owned by another son who was a local priest. Every winter when they came to Florida, the priest would arrange for home health care for his mother, through a doctor friend who would do him a favor. The hospital would provide the services until the mother went back North again in the spring. The spot on her buttocks had been there for years, and had never presented a problem in over ten years, she obviously needed no nursing care, she only wanted the aide to do the personal care and did not want to pay for it. Unfortunately, she had to claim some sort of problem which brought in the RN who then wrote for the aide. My visits were tolerated by the mother and son, and it became readily apparent that they could care less if I visited or not.

I decided early on that this was a challenge, and I was going to take the challenge to the limit on this one. From the office I called the manufacturer of skin care medications, and asked for their research department. I received a sales person on the line who specialized in helping nurses with special problems. I told him about the case I was seeing, and described that I felt the continual wetness of the mother was aggravating the area on her buttocks making it look like a wound. He understood the problem completely, and said that he had a new product that moisture, urine, anything could not penetrate through. He sent out several large tubes of the product for me to try and report back.

Armed with the new medication I went into combat with the spot on her ass. I squeezed some of the medication onto the spot and rubbed it all around the area, and on both cheeks of her ass. It looked like a white chalk but stuck to her ass like glue. I went into the bathroom with my gloves on and tried to wash the ointment off the gloves with soap and water, it would not budge, I could not wash this stuff off the gloves no matter how hard I tried. I immediately got a smile on my face as I felt that I was getting the upper hand on this case.

The aide seeing the mother, left me a note asking to talk to me about the case. I met with her and she asked me "what the hell did I put on the mother's ass" I explained the care I was providing, and she said "no matter how I tried I can't get that stuff off of the mother'. I said "don't try so hard, just do your normal care and let things take their course." She said "thanks" and said she would let the stuff stay there. Over a week went by and I continued to apply coat after coat of the salve to the mother. Neither the son or the mother took any interest whatsoever in what I was doing, as they both had been through various attempts at messing with her ass for ten years to no avail. They were smug in their security that they would go on as before and nothing I did would matter, they both thought "knock yourself out."

A little over a week later I did a thorough examination of the mother's ass and could not for the life of me find the spot on her skin. The skin was as soft and spot free as a baby's ass. I went out to the kitchen and told the son that I was ending the home health car and today would be the last visit for all services. The son was reading the newspaper at the time, and he put it down and looked like he was about to suffer a stroke. He stammered something unintelligible, and called the mother into the kitchen. He stood up, grabbed the mother and positioned her facing away from himself toward me. He abruptly pulled her fresh diaper down and went into a frenzy inspecting her ass. There was nothing to be found, he was dumbfounded. I presented him with the medication I had used and instructed him on the application of it and where to get the medication if he ran out. I filled out the chart, closed it out, and left.

I never returned to that condo, and the aide told me that she never went back either. I am sure that the agency reassigned another team to the case, but I couldn't verify it because I didn't know all the teams. The look on the son's face as he searched his mother's ass for that spot was worth a million dollars to me. I went on to promote that cream in dozens of other cases and it worked every time. That cream saved Medicare thousands and thousands of dollars. Of course, eliminating the fraud would help too.

THE CHEF

Seated in an overstuffed chair in the middle of the room

The next case was a patient that was discharged home because of an unverified lie to the case manager by the patient. The patient should have been placed into a nursing home to live as he was totally unable to care for himself in any way. I received the case as a new admission, who had been discharged the afternoon before my AM visit. The condo apartment was on the second floor of the complex and the front door was unlocked. I knocked and heard someone yell "come in." I entered and was greeted by a horrible shit smell hanging in the stuffy air inside the condo. Inside was a large gelatinous man seated in an overstuffed cloth chair in the middle of the room. As I approached, I found the source of the shit smell, he had defecated all over himself in the chair. It was a terrible mess, I asked him if he had been in that chair since his discharge, because I could see into the bedroom and it had not been occupied. He reported that he had been in the chair since discharge, so I decided to get to work and clean him up as we talked. I brought a kitchen chair next to him and covered it with a couple chucks. (disposable pads) I then helped him up into a standing position which was a joke because he could not stand at all. Finally, I was able to muscle him onto the kitchen chair, but it allowed the cloth chair to reek even worse. I had to get it out of the condo so I drug it out onto the patio and closed the door. I then got some soapy water and washed him as best as I could trying to move him side to side as I cleaned. Eventually I was able to move him after he was cleaned up, into another chair loaded with chucks that could be pulled out one by one if he messed again soon. As each was pulled out a clean one would be underneath and they were waterproof. I told him that he could not live there alone unable to care for himself or prepare food. He then reported that the next-door neighbor was going to take care of him. I went next door and knocked, an elderly man answered the door, and I asked him if he was responsible for caring for the man next door. The gentleman said that he knew him in passing, but that was all. I went back to the condo (lets call the patient the chef because he was a retired chef) of the chef and reported that he was lying to me. He then stated that his nephew was coming in today to take care of him. I asked for his name and cell phone number and called him, the nephew answered that he knew nothing about his uncle. This was becoming a problem very quickly, it was a dangerous situation all around, and I was going to resolve it now. I told the chef that I was going to 911 him back to the hospital to be placed from there into a nursing home. He retorted that he would refuse the 911 call and would not go back to the hospital, and he further would refuse to go to a nursing home. We had reached am impasse, I reported that I would not admit him to home health care because we were not able to provide the total care he needed, there is no way an aide could handle his bulk as he outweighed me by about 70 pounds and I weighed 200 lbs. Someone was going to get hurt trying to move his bulk without a hydraulic lift and several people to double team his care which a nursing home could provide. Then there was the shopping and food preparation and feeding issue which the chef was not even considering. I gave him one last chance, and he refused, so I left him and went back to the office to have a meeting with my supervisor about the chef. I related everything to her, and I heard later she assigned the chef to another team. I wish I was there to see the nurse when she walked through the door of that condo to do the admission. This story just illustrates the lengths home health will go to, to retain a patient so they can get the $$.

There is story after story about miscalculations made by family members when the decision has to be made if the patient is to be put into a nursing home or brought home to be taken care of there. Too many people unfamiliar with the care of an invalid, assume that they will be able to do it themselves. They don't realize that the nurse, aide or therapist perform their duties and go on to the next patient. What about the time when assist is not present, like all night. Wives say "I'll never put my husband in a nursing home, I couldn't do that to him." The wife is 110 lbs. and the husband is 6'2" and 235 lbs., who's kidding who, with her statement. I always stumbled onto these cases with the admission visit because it is the first contact outside the hospital.

I WANT HIM HOME
She would ruin her beautiful home

I went to a nice single home where a stroke patient paralyzed on the left side was discharged the day before. The house was occupied by a husband and wife only, no other person to help take care of the husband. The husband was in the bed and the wife was running around the house in a lather trying to figure how to toilet her husband who had indicated that he had to make a BM. I went to work right away getting the husband up on his one good leg only to find that he could barely stand on it, and not for long. I struggled to turn him at the bedside and move him into the bathroom. As soon as he was erect, he began to evacuate his bowels on the bedroom rug. He continued as we both struggled to get him into the toilet, leaving a trail behind us. I managed to get him seated on the toilet, but for the most part he had messed all over the floor and was just about done when he got seated. Now came the toughest part, which was to get him from the toilet to the living room, which is where his wife had picked out to deposit him. I cleaned him up and we managed to get him seated in the living room using a maximum effort on my part both holding him up and swinging his flaccid leg along as it wanted to drag behind him. There were no aids of any kind in the house, like a gait belt, as he was not admitted yet. The wife was busying herself trying to clean up the mess all over the white rugs but she had only succeeded in making a much bigger mess than she had originally. She was on her last nerve and whimpering when she came out of the bedroom. I asked to talk to her alone outside the home on the lawn. I knew she could not handle the husband, and in trying she would ruin her beautiful home, and that's what I told her. Her husband should have placement where she could visit with him all day if she wanted, but would be able to come home to rest at night. She knew she was in a pickle, but kept repeating that she would find a way to keep him home with GOD's help. I reinforced my advice to her stating that she needed either massive amounts of equipment brought in, or two strong men right away. I tried to impress on her that she was totally incapable of maintaining her husband at home the way things were. I advised her that if she was determined to have him home, she should admit him to a nursing home for the amount of time it took to retrofit the home for invalid care, and hire significant help. She kept saying that she would keep him home no matter what, ignoring my advice. I accomplished the admission, booked all the services and decided to let matters take their course. I tried to go back three days later, and the door was locked and no one was home, I never saw them again.

DONE RIGHT

Rarely had I seen such a wonderful arrangements

I only saw one home where the family had everything in hand. I had picked up this patient while the RN was on two weeks vacation. I enter a very nice home through the front door, and the interior was beautiful, everything was white with red accents. (they were Italian) A woman showed me to the bedroom where the patient was lying in a hospital bed watching a wall mounted tv. The patient was non-verbal due to advanced age and senility. The floor of the room was tiled in nice white vinyl floor tile, and there was a bureau against a white ceramic tiled wall. The bureau had everything necessary on it placed in the perfect position for easy use. There was a pneumatic lift tucked in the corner of the room with a selection of slings near it. I examined the patient, and she was clean and neat as a pin with no odor other than the pleasant smell of lotion. She was in an ideal situation and I was able to see to my tasks quite easily and it was a pleasure to work in such a well-thought-out situation. When I finished my visit, I stopped near the door to tell the family that rarely had I seen such a wonderful arrangement for a relative, and she would be very proud of their efforts if she knew what they had done. They thanked me, and I left to go on my rounds, but I was in admiration of the retrofitting they had done to the room, it was absolutely perfect for providing care at home.

The retrofit was inexpensive and was done by the people themselves using a little thought and planning. It was a better arrangement than you could find in an extended care facility, cleaner, better lit, and the patient was in excellent shape for someone immobile, and the care was outstanding.

TWO HUSBANDS

Procedure after procedure and test after test

We all make choices in life, some are good and some are bad. We don't find out whether they are good or bad until the outcome is decided. This is the story of two different choices, and two different outcomes, you pick which one was good or which one was bad, I have my opinion.

Two couples lived in an assisted living home, they were both across the hall from each other, and were very good friends. They did things together, ate many meals together, and thought the world of each other. After living there for eight years, both of the husbands received bad news during their routine physicals. Each was notified that they had to undergo some very crucial testing for prostate cancer. Now, there are two types of prostate cancer, one is rapid growing and is deadly, and the other is very slow growing, and most patients with this type usually die from something else before the cancer gets them. The testing was accomplished, and both husbands were told that they had the rapid growing kind.

Both husbands had a decision to make, to treat the disease aggressively, and try to gain more time before the disease takes them, or refuse treatment and live with the disease as best he can, and let what comes without treatment. One husband and wife decided to take every treatment available in hopes that they would have a lot more time together until the end. The other couple decided to refuse treatment and just live whatever time they had left together. The husband that decided to be treated, began by having an IV port placed in his chest. He went to the Urologist and had a series of seed implants placed into the prostate gland. (this required accessing the prostate through the rectum, and stabbing the prostate with a needle to implant radioactive seeds) He continued to go through procedure after procedure and test after test. Some of the procedures caused a great deal of discomfort, and some made him very ill. At times he was unable to eat, and spent a significant amount of time in bed recovering from the hospital and doctor visits.

The second husband who denied all treatment quickly booked a cruise while he felt well. When he returned from the cruise, he still felt pretty good, so he took a trip out west to a spa where he received a special homeopathic diet, massages, hot treatments in a native American sweat lodge. He enjoyed it so well that he stayed an additional week. He returned home, and decided that two alcoholic drinks a day would make him feel better, so he had them. Eventually he received palliative care from his doctor to include pain medications, and others to assist him until the end. He spent the last month of his life reading a few books he always wanted to read, and fell asleep reading them in his favorite chair. He died at home with hospice care and his wife in attendance.

The husband that took all the treatments died two months after the other, however, he spent all the time at home, most of it suffering from either treatment, doctor visits, scans, or other procedures related to his disease. His wife agreed that he started as a big strong guy, and by the end she didn't recognize him anymore, and his passing was a blessing.

Both wives are still friends, each with their own memories to cherish.

FEED ME BABY, FEED ME

There she was dressed as a nurse

Many patients who have suffered a stroke, are able to function pretty well in the home environment. Physical therapy can work wonders if the paralysis is not too severe. However, in some cases the patients relearn tasks to a high degree and function well. This is the case of an elderly gentleman who suffer such a stroke, did well, but was left with an inability to swallow correctly. When you can't swallow correctly, you usually receive a feed tube placed through the stomach wall, and liquid nourishment is poured down the tube into the stomach.

The liquid nourishment is specially prepared for the patient based on recommendations provided by a nurse specially educated in these preparations. Usually, patients do very well on the liquid nourishment, which is either poured into the tube, or the patient is placed on a metered pump. Once the required amount has been ingested, the patient tucks the feed tube into his clothing, and goes about his business until the next feed.

I was sent to this gentleman's home to train someone in how to conduct the feedings and how to care for the feed tube placed into the stomach through the skin. The gentleman lived in a large home where he was attended by his wife and an extended family. When I arrived, I asked the family to select someone to receive the training, because my number of visits for training were very limited. The patient's wife said she would do the feedings, so I went right to work with her instruction. I went through everything, and she voiced that she understood, and was very eager to conduct the feedings. After several successful evolutions, I left advising her that I would return on the next day to continue to monitor her and reinforce the training.

The following day, I showed up, and the wife had an area set aside in the house looking very sterile, with everything she thought she could ever need. And there she was, dressed as a nurse, complete with a store-bought uniform, with all the trimmings. She had more shit on her than I had, and she was ready to get the job done. She went right to work on her husband, setting everything up and doing the job as good as anyone could do it. I could see from the husbands face, that he was a little disgusted with the big nurse act put on by his wife. I decided that I would make one more visit the next day and that would be all. I never got to go back again. The husband decided regardless of the swallowing issue, he was going to eat dinner with the family, come what may. If he choked to death on the food, so be it, he was not going through this giant feeding fiasco with his costumed wife, and that was that.

NOT LIKE ON TV

While calling the code he reverted to his native language

Most people get their view of what goes on in a hospital from T.V. shows like; ER or Grey's Anatomy. If a cardiac arrest occurs, there are residents and attending physicians who work the code. In my thirty-eight years of working in nursing, I have never seen a doctor insert an I.V., do chest compressions, defibrillate a patient, or insert an airway. During a code, if a doctor is available, he will run the code (give orders). Once I was on a cardiac unit where we had two codes going at the same time. The ER physician came up on the floor and ran one code, and the nursing supervisor ran the other. If memory serves me right, there were two other physicians on the unit at that time, neither one volunteered to help. During a code, nurses and the respiratory therapist will perform the functions of a code (insert an I.V., an airway, shock the patient and give drugs). Only if you are in a teaching hospital are there residents in house. In the evenings at most hospitals, the only physician in house is the ER doctor.

While working on the cardiology unit at night, in a small hospital, in a neighboring county, one of the patients went into cardiac arrest. The patient was unresponsive, and the telemetry rhythm showed pulse less V-Tach. Pulse less V-Tach is where the ventricles of the heart are beating rapidly, but without enough force to push blood throughout the body. A code was called, and the ER physician came up to the unit. The ER doctor was from Eastern Europe and spoke English with an accent. While calling the code he reverted to his native tongue, a language that none of the nurses understood. This is not uncommon for people who are bilingual and under stress to start speaking in their native language. Luckily the charge nurse started giving orders. The rest of the team ignored the doctor and followed the instructions given by the charge nurse. The funny thing was, he continued to give orders oblivious to the fact no one was paying attention to him.

I guarantee you would never see anything like what I described on a television show. Thanks to her knowledge and professionalism the patient managed to survive, which is unusual. Unlike T.V., in the real world only 30% of hospital patients survive a code. After the patient was resuscitated, his primary physician and cardiologist were informed, and he was moved to the I.C.U. A week later he was discharged.

A GOOD CODE

There was no noticeable brain damage

Most codes DO NOT have a good outcome. This story involves three good codes on the same person, a thirty-three year old man. The man was out in his yard when he was stung by a bee. The man was allergic to bee stings. He walked into his house and collapsed on the kitchen floor. Luckily, his wife and neighbor were in the kitchen at the time. The wife called 9/11, while the neighbor performed C.P.R. The paramedics were able to restore circulation and transported him to the E.R. In the E.R., he coded a second time. The E.R. staff managed to resuscitated him and move him to the I.C.U. After two days in the I.C.U., he was transferred to the telemetry floor. On the telemetry floor, he coded again and was resuscitated for the third time in less than a week. He was returned to the I.C.U. The patient's doctor told his wife that he will probably suffer from brain damage. After three days in the I.C.U. he was transferred back to the telemetry floor. He spent another three days, there before being discharged home. Upon being discharged, there was no noticeable brain damage. The patient's speech was clear; he could walk and feed himself. His memory was good.

A month after he was discharged he returned to the hospital to thank the staff for saving his life. I asked him about his mentation. He said he had no problems except for seizures. He was able to control the seizure by drinking hemp smoothies. He seemed a little embarrassed telling me this, and went out of his way to assure me that he was not a drug addict, and he had never used illicit drugs before his code. I told him thought never crossed my mind. I also told him that I thought he looked and sounded really good for someone who coded three times. I am glad he was able to get back to living a normal life.

Finally, I informed him that in the sixties the U.S Department of Public Health experimented with marijuana as a treatment for seizure patients. What I understand is that the experiment proved successful. I was not sure why the experiment was terminated. I also told him that until 1937 marijuana was legally sold in American pharmacies. Lastly, I told him, if hemp smoothies were preventing his seizure and he was not suffering any side effects he probably should continue. I guess he is doing well because I never saw him in the hospital again.

50 CENTS IS STILL SOMETHING
Physical assaults are very common

After working fourteen years as a R.N., I became worried about what would happen if I could not work anymore, as a nurse. For example, if I hurt my back (which is a common injury in nursing). It is very difficult for R.N.s to get any kind of disability. You are usually told, "You are a R.N. you can get a sit down job." This is what happened to my wife, when she was denied disability after a back injury. She was told by her physician she could not lift more than twenty-five pounds. After great difficulty, she was able to get a job with an insurance company. Also, a classmate of mine from nursing school was told the same thing and was denied disability after her back injury. She was finally able to get disability when she was diagnosed with breast cancer. I decided I needed a plan B, so, I decided to get a master's degree in library science as plan B. I figured even if I was in a wheelchair I could work as a reference librarian.

After graduation, I was hired by the local community college as a part-time medical librarian. My starting salary was $25.00/hour. I had been working at the same hospital for seventeen years and my base pay was only $25.50/hour. I was pleasantly surprised by my first day working as a librarian. I was treated with respect. Nobody yelled at me, and I was not physically assaulted. Physical assaults on nurses are very common, according to the U.S. Department of Labor nurses are the third most likely group to be assaulted on the job. (the first is prison guards and the second being police officers) People thanked me, this almost never happens in nursing. After completing my shift, I did not feel beat up, which is the usual case in nursing. In fact, I felt so good I went bicycle riding after work.

The next day I was working as a nurse. I was helping another nurse get her patient from the bathroom back to bed. Her patient was a forty year old male alcoholic who was suffered from cirrhosis and his skin was yellow. While getting him back to bed the man urinated and defecated on the floor, then he collapsed. We lowered him to the floor, I checked for breathing and a pulse and there was none, so we called a code. With my knees in urine I proceeded to do CPR. While doing chest compressions, I thought this is why they pay me 50 cents an hour more to work here.

ALL ON ONE FLOOR

She was in full contact with the birds

Much of the work I did as a nurse was to work for a nursing agency. In fact, I worked for three nursing agencies at the same time for over two years. In order to work continuously I booked my work in the following manner. I would start with day shift usually 7AM to 7pm, if I got no morning call for an assignment, I would book the 3-11 shift. If I got no call for 3-11 I would book 7PM to 7AM and finally I would book 11-7 shift. In over two years I only missed two days work using this system. Working agency allowed me to have the independence to have days off that I really needed, and not be at the whim of a nursing supervisor. It also furnished me with funds that were in excess of a fully scheduled nursing job, because agency type work usually paid more. Agencies were very aggressive in placing their personnel anywhere that they were qualified for, which included some very interesting assignments. The variety in agency nursing was not everyone's cup of tea, but it enabled the nurse to add many talents that they would not otherwise be exposed to.

I was working agency at a local hospital during the 3-11 shift and had a very eclectic group of patients that were very interesting in many ways. Never before had I encountered such a group that I had not been exposed to before. All of them tragic in their own way.

The first was a middle-aged patient that had been admitted to the floor several days before, because she was to undergo testing to determine the source of the symptoms she was experiencing. I was in her room doing vital signs when the physician came in to inform her of the diagnosis the tests revealed. I knew something was up, because he physician looked like he was very upset and didn't want to be there under any circumstances. I finished my work and left the doctor and patient alone, and went on to my next patient.

Later in the evening when I returned to the room the woman was very upset and it was not hard to notice that she had been crying. She seemed to be finished crying and was getting very angry, and asked me if she could talk to me just to vent a little. I went over to a chair at the bedside and sat down to listen to her and told her to tell me whatever was bothering her. She started by recounting the conversation she had with the doctor. He informed her that her tests revealed that she had a very advanced case of ovarian cancer that had spread to many other organs in her body. She asked the doctor what could be done to fight the ovarian cancer, and he said that nothing presently available in medicine could cure this advanced disease. She continued by asking the doctor how she could have advanced ovarian cancer when she had a hysterectomy (removal of her ovaries) many years before. The doctor informed her that the surgeon had done a partial hysterectomy on one side and left a piece of an ovary so she would not have to take estrogen replacement therapy. The remaining piece of her ovary was now malignant and had spread to most of her organs thereby eliminating the possibility of successful treatment. At that point there was nothing left to say and the doctor asked if she wanted to return home, or did she feel too unwell, in which case he would request placement for her through the social worker. She said that she would make that decision after she talked with her family members.

I expressed condolences to her about the diagnosis, and prepared to make my exit. She in her anger said she could kill the original surgeon for leaving the piece of ovary in there. She said she never knew what the surgeon was going to do, she never had a consultation where options were explained in full to her.

This did not surprise me at all because many many times I had followed a surgeon's instructions and obtained a surgical permit and had the patient sign it on the doctor's behalf. It was always the doctor's job to do that not the nurse. The doctor is fully responsible to explain to the patient, all the issues surrounding the surgery including everything that can go wrong. The patient should hear everything from the doctor before the surgical permit is presented for signature. I have had to substitute my knowledge for his frequently when I am ordered by the doctor to have the patient sign the permit. The patients almost always forget to ask the doctor pertinent questions especially when they are in the room alone and when the doctor arrives unannounced. Some nurses are better at explanations than others, and the patient is entitled to the best explanation possible.

THE BIRDS
Stay out of further contact with birds

Working on the same floor on the same day I encountered a male patient in his early 70's who had his daughter in the room with him. They were both very friendly, and the daughter volunteered that she had been a patient several years ago, and in fact was in the very same bed her father now occupied. They were both laughing about the coincidence when I went into the room to introduce myself and take a set of vital signs. Again, the father and daughter had more in common than they knew.

The daughter owned a home with a large screened structure at the rear of the house. The structure was attached to the home and could be accessed through a set of sliding doors to an open patio inside the screened area. She operated a business in the screened area, she was a bird breeder. She raised several types rare birds the largest group was a parakeet called a Sun Conure.

She related that she was depending on her father for supervision and care of the birds in the enclosure. She had been hospitalized many times for lung ailments related to her business. Repeated contact with bird droppings, shed feathers, and dead birds can cause a lung disease called histoplasmosis and she had contracted it many times in her business. On her last admission to the hospital she had been informed by the doctor that she had developed permanent damage to both lungs from the continued bouts of disease and she should stay out of further contact with birds.

Now that her father was ill, she was again in full contact with the birds going against the orders of her doctor. I went out to the chart to examine why her father was admitted to the hospital. The chart revealed that the father was diagnosed with the same illness as the daughter. Evidently he could not take the concentrated exposure to birds and their waste either. It seems that if they are smart, they both should find another line of work. The father related that once in a while he would get a parrot or cockatoo for free. Birds that escape from their owners would fly around searching for other similar birds to live with. He would find a lone bird walking around on top of the screened structure looking for a way to get inside. He would place food at a particular spot and the bird would eventually walk into an air lock to get the food. He would shut the outer door and open an inner door, and a free bird was in with the rest.

Exotic pets can be a problem for humans. Not all exotic pets have been cultured (swabs taken from their mouths and other parts and grown in petri dishes to ascertain what organisms are present that might harm humans) like domestic dogs and cats have. Every organism living on a dog or cat has been cultured by science numerous times, so we know everything they carry in their mouths, claws or nails, and in their feces and urine. Cats are more of a problem because they can transmit a bacteria to a human which causes an infection called cat scratch fever. It is transmitted by licking, fleas biting a human that have lived on a cat, and scratching with their claws or biting with their teeth.

Time to mention about preschool children and dogs brought to hospitals to see patients. Some people are just dumb and there is no way to fix dumb. Preschool children do not have complete immune systems. They should not be exposed to all of the illnesses present in a building full of sick and dying humans. Nurses have a difficult time being exposed to these diseases, and they have had every immunization available, and a full history of exposure to all of the childhood diseases. Even nurses contract illnesses that patients have brought into the hospital, so imagine the risk a baby or small child assumes while visiting an adult. So, you say "but my grandfather is in CCU with a heart attack he isn't sick so we can visit him without exposing ourselves to a disease." That is the biggest load of bullshit I have ever heard. Thousands of people have died in that bed, and the room has been cleaned up by a $5.00 per hour Mexican. As for dogs or other "comfort pets" being brought to the hospital, nurses don't take kindly to this, even if they are pet owners at home. Pets come in off the street, lick things, walk on bedclothes, sit on bedclothes, may have flea's, ticks, worms, and many other organisms living in their fur. It is risky to say the least, and should be avoided by any sane person.

NO SAFE DRUGS

Limbs are surgically sliced open

The next patient I saw that evening had a problem that I had not encountered before. He was a young man in his early twenties, with his family sitting in the room with him. I had to do his vital signs on his leg because his arms and one leg were bandaged. He was admitted with a self-inflicted problem that might kill him. The chart revealed the problem, which was related to taking drugs. Evidentially, he had been a recreational illicit drug user, and, wanting a high, had acquired some pills from a street corner source. With these type of purchases you get no instruction on the oral dose, other than the information provided by the idiot seller. Of course, one idiot to another, this is just fine, so he took the drugs home and at a selected time took the medications. He tried to rise up from a sitting position in a chair and passed out on the floor collapsing with parts of both arms under his body, and one leg under the other.

A normal person asleep would move every so often to allow blood to perfuse any area that had reduced supply from laying on it. In this fellows case, he was in a drug induced coma and lay on his extremities for an extended time without relieving the crushing weight and allowing the tissues to "breathe." He was found on the floor, after he did not answer the phone or door bell the next day. He had spent an extended time laying in one position without moving at all. The rescue squad was called, and he was admitted to the hospital suffering from a problem identified as Rhabdomyolysis. This is a disease where your skeletal muscles have died and the resulting damaged tissues flood into the blood stream and block the kidneys with waste product from the ruined tissues. The patient needs to have their kidneys flushed repeatedly by placing a dialysis access in their neck area and putting them on a dialysis machine because their kidneys have shut down. Additionally, the affected limbs are surgically sliced open to drain the poisonous byproduct coming from the tissues into bandages to help get it out of the body instead of through the bloodstream. Both of his arms and one leg were sliced wide open to drain. These were man made wounds which would be closed surgically at a later date when or if the kidneys recovered and the full extent of damage to the limbs had been assessed. Tissue repair by the body would be quite extensive, and it was unknown at the time what permanent effects he would suffer for the rest of his life. There was not much a nurse could do in this case because he was taken to dialysis on a schedule and spent hours there running his blood through the machine to flush it. His wound dressings would be changed while he was there. I felt sorry for him just because he had no idea what he would do to himself when he swallowed those pills.

MERRY CHRISTMAS, STUPID

It is always difficult setting up home care before holidays

Working one Christmas Eve as a home health care coordinator, I received a referral to set up a forty something female with home health care. The woman had an abscess on her lower leg. It seems she had a bug bite that she scratched and a MRSA (a nasty penicillin resistant germ) infection developed. This is not unusual in Florida. The services the woman needed were daily dressing changes and I.V. Vancomycin, twice a day. Vancomycin is one of the few medications that are effective against MRSA.

In setting up this woman for home care, I faced two problems. The first was it was Christmas Eve. It is always difficult setting up home care before holidays, with Christmas being the worse. The reason is, most nurses want the day off, to spend the holiday with their families, so home health care agencies do not have the staff to begin accepting new patients. The second problem was, the woman was a Medicaid patient. Medicaid is a joint Federal/State program. Benefits vary from state to state. Some states are very generous; Florida is not one of those states. In Florida, Medicaid pays only $29.95 for a home care nursing visit. It costs a home care agency $60.00 per nursing visit, so with each nursing visit the agency will lose $30.05. Most home health care agencies are for profit businesses, thus they will not accept Florida Medicaid patients. In my area of Florida, there were four non-profit home care agencies and they would accept only a limited number of Medicaid patients.

The first non-profit agency I called said they would accept the patient, but they could not send a nurse out until the evening of Christmas day. I was elated. I informed the patient that I had found an agency and they could begin her home care tomorrow evening. After receiving her morning dose of Vancomycin on Christmas day, she could be discharged. Instead of being happy, the woman angrily said to me "do you know what day it is?" I responded "yes Christmas Eve." She said "that is right. I have a party to go to." I then told her I was sorry, but this is the best I could offer her and left the room.

First thing in the morning Christmas day, I went to see the patient to make a copy of the final discharge orders to send to the home health care agency. When I discovered the patient was not in her room, I asked the charge nurse where she was, and was told last night she left AMA (against medical advice) with her picc line intact (a picc line is a central line used for patients getting long term antibiotics) I returned to my office and informed the agency they would not be getting the patient.

Two days later, I received a telephone call from the patient. She wanted to know when she was going to get her home health care. I informed her by going AMA she negated my responsibility of setting up home care. She told me her picc-line was still in place and wanted to know what she should do. I told her to call her doctor and maybe his office could setup home care for her. While giving her instructions, what was going through my mind was this person was both selfish and stupid. In order to have some fun, she was willing to expose everyone at the party to an infectious disease and she also missed three days of vital treatment for a serious bout of MRSA.

THE ONLY ALTERNATIVE
Harrington rods are a one way street

This was a sorry case admitted to the hospital for an unknown reason, because there was nothing anyone could do for her except to try and make her as comfortable as possible, and that was impossible as the physicians would soon find out.

The patient was approximately 85 or so years old. She was all twisted and folded up by arthritis, and multiple ailments like Osteoporosis. She was so contorted that she could not lay flat in bed, her posture made her look like she was trying to sit up in bed, but she was not. There was also a massive internal problem which probably caused her admission, she had a Harrington rod placed when she was a young girl, and now due to her spine problems it had ripped loose. Harrington rods are installed when people are young to prevent the spine from growing crooked. There are several issues which call for these rods to be used, but we won't get into them here. In this lady's case the top attaching point had broken loose and the rod was pushing against her skin behind the shoulder trying to force its way out. She was in excruciating pain to the point of not being able to eat or sleep, just laying there moaning and crying.

Physicians had examined the patient and her x-rays and determined that she was not a candidate for surgery because she could not take the anesthesia, nor could they unravel the lower attaching point of the rod to remove it, Harrington rods are a one way street. Of course, this put her in a terrible spot, because the pain associated with the misplaced rod was getting worse each hour as it forced its way up and out of her body. She was on constant pain medication which seemed to do her little good.

Her hospital based (teaching hospital) young physician went in to explain everything to her about the decisions that had been made. She was a hopeless case, and they were considering transferring her to a nursing home with lots of pain med orders to let her live out her life there. To put it mildly the patient was scared shitless. When the young doctor came out of the room, he was very upset for her, and after some reflection gave me an order for medication. He instructed me to "give her 8 mg of morphine IV for pain." I was surprised because I knew that 8 mg would put her down permanently. I remarked to the doctor that the dose would kill the patient, and he responded, "either you give it, or I will." That also surprised me, but I resolved to give it as he wrote the order in the chart. I signed out the dose and went into the room and confronted the patient. She was terrified (at least that was the look on her face) and I told her that the doctor had ordered something that would make her pain go away, and without further ado, pushed the dose into her IV line and left the room to dispose of part of the syringe. (morphine doses require a 2 part syringe, one half you throw away and the other is reused for subsequent doses) I waited several minutes, saw another patient, and returned to the room , and the patient had fallen into a deep sleep and died on the spot. I notified the physician who was still on the floor, and he pronounced the patient. He left the floor, and I went back to work until the end of the shift. Two hospital aides cleaned the woman, placed her in a shroud tagged her toe, and shipped her off to the morgue. It was all in a day's work, but until recently it bothered me immensely. I had the opportunity recently to talk to another retired RN who heard the story and said it was the kindest thing I could have done for the woman, but I still think about it.

THE VIETNAM VET
He lived in a trailer and received a disability

Section by Vince Frattaruolo

We use to get a regular patient on the floor who was a Vietnam vet. He suffered from C.O.P.D. and angina. He was also missing a leg. The man suffered from nightmares. In order to get a night's sleep, we would have to give him 30 mg of Restoril and 5 mg of Valium. When he was not in the hospital he lived in a trailer and received a disability check from the V.A. He never spoke of family or friends and no one visited him in the hospital. Increasingly the man was unable to take care of himself. The doctor and social workers wanted him to go to a V.A. nursing home, but for some reason he refused. Instead he went back to his trailer, with home health care. When the home health care nurse made his visit, he found the veteran dead. The patient was on the floor with the blinds on top of him. What we think happened was he was in distress grabbed the blinds and tried to stand up. The blinds could not hold the patient's weight and he collapsed with the blinds falling on top of him. Historians will tell you that the Vietnam War ended in 1975, but for this veteran the war ended in 1998 with his death.

Section by John Bankhead

I was working home health, and one of my morning visits was in a run-down old trailer park. In a trailer close to the entrance lived a Vietnam war veteran with one leg. In the morning he was always my first visit, and he was always sitting facing the door in his favorite chair. He had a slew of medical problems and he looked like he would lose his one good leg in the not to distant future. The leg showed very bad circulation problems, and was horribly discolored below the knee. He was always a jolly fellow, and he enjoyed talking to me while I did my assigned examinations, and treatments. One of his great joys was eating spaghetti that he fixed every day for supper, he had that dish down pat, and once in a while a male friend in the same trailer park would come and have a bowl of spaghetti with him.

On this particular morning, I parked in front of his unit, gathered my equipment and medical bag and climbed the metal steps to the trailer. I never knocked because he couldn't answer the door anyway, and I was instructed to come in because he knew I was coming as I had been for weeks. When I opened the door, I was surprised that he was not in his usual chair facing the door. I just assumed that he was in the bathroom, so I sat my things down on a chuck I had laid out, and called for him. There was no answer, so I went into the hall and knocked on the bathroom door, still no answer. At this point I suspected that I was going to find something all home care nurses dread, a body. I approached the bedroom and saw a messed-up bed but no occupant. When I entered the room all the way I saw a pale arm extended up toward the window with a venetian bling cord wrapped around the hand several times, and the blinds pulled all the way to the top of the window. I walked around the bed, and there he was on the floor dead. He evidently tried to get out of bed on his one good leg and fell between the bed and the wall pinning himself beyond his ability to get back up. He obviously struggled to rise, exhausting his ability to provide enough oxygen to his brain and asphyxiated. He was a well known lung patient, and his diseased lungs could not provide enough oxygen especially in his compressed space, and with his struggles to rise up to his feet, or foot.

I called 911 and reported the death and asked for the police to come and investigate the death to rule out foul play. I also called the office to report the same thing, and to have any other therapies cancelled so they wouldn't come to an empty trailer to visit a dead patient. After the police arrived, I gave them a business card with my information on it, and left to visit my next case which was only about 10 blocks away.

BETTER OFF DEAD

The prognosis was not very good

Unlike what you see on T.V. most people do not survive a cardiac arrest. The national average is 7.5%. Even if you survive, your quality of life may not be very good, you might be better off dead. When working on the telemetry floor I received a patient from the I.C.U. who had suffered a cardiac arrest at home. The patient was a seventy-five year old male, who complained of chest pain. His girlfriend called 9/11. By the time the paramedics arrived, he was unresponsive, did not have a pulse and was not breathing. The paramedics immediately went to work and coded him. They continued the code while the man was taken to the E.R. The E.R. staff worked on him for forty-five minutes, before circulation was restored. He was then moved to I.C.U. He spent four days in I.C.U. and was then transferred to my unit.

When I got him, he was confused and was attempting to pull out his I.V. lines, so he had to be restrained (his arms tied down). His speech was inarticulate and he did not know he was in a hospital or the year. He could not feed himself, so he had to be fed.

If no oxygen gets to the brain (oxygen is carried by blood and if a person goes into cardiac arrest there is no circulation) brain damage could be the result. For some reason, he also needed kidney dialysis. Before his cardiac arrest, he had no history of renal insufficiency. After three days on the telemetry floor, he was transferred to a nursing home, for rehab.

Two weeks later I received the patient back from the nursing home. He was still confused and inarticulate, he was no long on dialysis, but he did have a large decubitus ulcer on his coccyx. Among laymen it is known as a bed sore.

This wound was deep and went to the bone. This condition happens when the patient is left in one position too long, or is left lying in feces or urine. Treating this type of patient with a decubitus ulcer is difficult. In order to heal the wound the patient needs to be well nourished. This is difficult if the person cannot feed himself. Feeding a patient takes valuable time from a busy schedule. He needs to be kept clean, turned frequently (every two hours). Dressing changes were ordered every shift.

A wound culture was done and the wound was positive for MRSA (staphylococcus resistant bacteria). It was decided the wound need long term antibiotics (six weeks) so a picc line (central line in a larger blood vessel) was placed. Two weeks later he was returned to his nursing home. From past experience, I can tell that his prognosis is not very good. His last days will be spent shuttling back and forth from nursing home to hospital. At some point, he will probably end up with a pneumonia which is common with these immobile patients. If he does not die from another heart attack, he will probably expire due to Sepsis. Sepsis is known to layman as blood poisoning. It is a severe infection which leads to multiple organ damage and frequently death. It is common among debilitated elderly people who all have compromised immune systems. Patients like this one soak up money and resources like a sponge, all to no avail, nothing can be done to resurrect their prior life.

CAN THEY SELL IT ALL?

Flatware salt and pepper shakers and sugar bowls

When I first started nursing, I was on a telemetry floor of a local hospital when the King of the Gypsies was admitted on the next wing. I had never seen a gypsy community anywhere near where I was living, but there were several palm reader shops nearby with neon signs in the window offering to tell your fortune. Most of the nurses on the floor thought of it as a novelty, with the patient's room, and hallway near the room loaded with visitors. The male nurses thought it was fun because of the scantily clad young women all over the place. Night and day there were no less than twenty or thirty gypsies congregating near the room where the King was holding court.

Being a car nut, I loved walking through the parking lot on my way out of the building because there was a conglomeration of expensive cars in the lot parked there by the gypsy visitors. There were any number of Mercedes, Jaguar, custom SUV's, and custom Cadillac's, they put the doctor's cars to shame. The visitors tried hard to stay there 24 hours a day, but eventually the hospital was able to get them to leave several hours after visitor hours were over.

By the third day, the nurses noticed that IV poles were in exceptional short supply, we could not find them in the usual place. I looked in all the patient's rooms and the supply room and only found two, and there were many more than two usually on the floor. The next thing that went missing was chairs. Chairs in areas of the hospital where there were waiting rooms full of chairs began to diminish leaving empty spaces in the row where chairs were. Then the cafeteria was running out of flatware, salt and pepper shakers, and sugar bowls. Then the framed prints on the walls somehow left the building. Then phones were missing from the walls leaving the plugs hanging connected to thin air.

The codes on the drug supplies were changed repeatedly like never before, to prevent an observer from gaining access to the cabinet when the RN's were busy. Everyone was watching, but we never saw anyone take anything, but things continued to get out of the building. We remarked that they had better find some way to get the King discharged while we still had a building left. After a while the staff thought it funny waiting to see what would be targeted next by the thieves. We would sit together during our breaks or lunch sharing observations about what was stripped from the building today.

Eventually, the King was gone, and the hospital had to reorder everything that "got legs" and things settled down to the mundane things we had known before. We could never find out how things were smuggled out of the building despite cameras, security and door locks, but whoever did it they were a master at it.

2 QUESTIONS AND 5 STORIES
They would pick eight bad choices and two good

In nursing classes law and ethics was taught by a man who had an M.D. and a J.D. (Doctor of Jurisprudence). He had a legal practice that specialized in medical malpractice. He was an adjunct professor (part-time professor) the only course he taught was law and ethics for nurses. He would use the Socratic Method to teach (asking questions rather than lecturing). Some of the questions left the class speechless. One question he asked the class was, if a woman comes into my office and has a miscarriage, I have to fill out a death certificate. If she comes into my office, and has an abortion I take the fetus place it in a medical waste bag. Why don't I have to fill out a death certificate? No one could give him an answer.

Another question he asked was whether Greg Louganis should have told the doctor who sutured his head that he had A.I.D.S. Louganis was competing in diving at the 1988 Olympics. While making a dive he hit his head against the diving board and suffered a laceration that need to be sutured. The class responded with a no, the doctor should be using universal precautions and Louganis might lose endorsements if sponsors knew he had A.I.D.S. The professor responded what about the other divers. The class stated that chlorine in the water should have killed the virus. The professor said "I want everybody in this class who would be willing to jump in a pool after Greg Louganis bled in it to raise your hand." Not a single hand went up.

One clinical rotation I had to do for public health, was Women at Risk. Women at Risk, was a public health program targeting pregnant woman who were at risk for complications.   In order to be part of the program, the woman had to be under twenty-one years of age, over thirty-five, or did not possess a high school diploma. The program consisted of a public health nurse going to the pregnant woman's residence and informing them what programs were available (Medicaid and Food Stamps). The nurse also made sure that the patient had a doctor following her throughout the pregnancy. Finally, the nurse was to make sure the woman was eating nutritious meals, and was not doing anything that would harm her health or that of the baby.

UNSUPERVISED TEENS
She was afraid of going to jail

The first house the public health nurse and I visited was built in either the 1930' or 40's (which meant it was well built). There was garbage on the front lawn and the screening was ripped off the front porch windows. The nurse knocked on the door and this teenage boy with metallic orange hair answered the door. The nurse informed the teenager who we were there to see, and gave the pregnant woman's legal name. The teenager responded she does not live here. The nurse said "we are from the Public Health Department and this is the address she gave." The kid said oh you mean, (blank) and gave the woman's nickname. He called for her and she invited us into the house. We sat down in the living room right by a bag of garbage. As I looked around, I thought to myself, if they cleaned this place it would be a nice place, the walls were plaster, the floors were real wood, and there was a fire place in the living room.

The patient was a nineteen year old, who was being paid to take care of two teenage boys by their parents. The woman also did day labor. She had been pregnant once before and was pressured into having an abortion. She decided that she wanted to keep this baby. She did not want us to put the name of the baby's father in our chart because she was afraid of going to jail. It turned out that the fifteen year old boy with metallic orange hair impregnated her. While we were discussing the pregnancy with the woman, the father sat nearby, with head phones on listening to music. The woman also told us, that she took out a $4,000 student loan and enrolled in the nurse's aide program at Florida Metropolitan University (a non-accredited for profit school that has gone out of business). When we left the house, I turned to the public health nurse and asked "what is going on here. We have a fifteen year old kid who impregnated a woman and he does not know her legal name. She takes out a $4,000 loan to become a nurse's aide. The county vocational technical school charges only $400 for the nurse's aide course or she can go to a hospital, and they will train her for free and guarantee her a job when she graduates." She responded "what you see here is my typical client. If you gave them a piece of paper with ten good choices on one side and ten bad choices on the other, they would pick eight bad choices and two good.

MONEY WAS NO PROBLEM

She now qualifies for social services

The next house we visited was in a middle-class neighborhood. We pulled into the driveway and parked in front of a two car garage. The doorbell was answered by two attractive women; a mother and her sixteen year old pregnant daughter. I entered the house and sunk down six inches on a plush carpet. I looked around and noticed a huge wide screen T.V. I also saw a built in screened in swimming pool. The public nurse was told by the girl's mother that the girl already has signed up for Medicaid and Food Stamps. As we left the house, I turned to the nurse and asked "these people do not look poor. How can she get Medicaid and Food Stamps"? The nurse responded "if your teenage daughter gets pregnant out of wedlock you can emancipate her. Now she is not your responsibility, and since she has no income, she now qualifies for social services."

Our last visit was to an apartment of a pregnant thirty-eight year old, who abandoned her house, husband and two children to run off with a nineteen year old construction worker. I thought to myself, in ten years her looks will fade and she will probably be abandoned by the construction worker, if they last that long. I also thought the class should be changed from "Women at Risk" to taxpayer funded bad choices. Women over 35 have an increased risk of both Down's Syndrome and stillbirth. Risk of Downs syndrome are about 1 in 200 births taken to term in older mothers. A large portion of Downs Syndrome babies do not live to full term. Old maternal eggs present a host of other problems to older mothers and the babies who come from those eggs.

PUBLIC HEALTH
Where are your American patients

One of the courses I took in nursing school was "Public Health." Like most nursing courses it consisted of two parts: lecture and clinical. Lectures are a classroom lessons while clinicals are on the job training. For "Public Health" I was sent to the local public health clinic. One of the programs at the clinic was Well Child. Well Child consisted of physicals and treatment of minor aliments; colds, ear aches, and sore throats. Almost all of the patients were from Mexico and Central America. Out of a hundred children, only one was an American. There was a woman who was interpreting for the patients and their families. I first assumed she worked for the health department. After talking to her, I found out I was wrong, she was a freelancer. Every day she came to the health department, and would charge the illegal immigrants five to ten dollars to interpret for them. With this help, they would understand what the doctors and nurses were telling them. I asked the interpreter, where the parents of these children worked. She responded that they worked for local businesses and contractors, she further stated that they received less than minimum wage and no benefits. I asked one of the public health nurses "where are your American patients."

She responded, "if you are an American citizen or a legal immigrant, you are put on a Medicaid H.M.O. and you see a private doctor, but if you're an illegal immigrant you can't be put on Medicaid, so you come to the public health department."

Several thoughts went through my mind, first we will never end illegal immigration because the contractors and businessmen are making too much money off of it.

Also, eventually the illegals will someday get amnesty, and become citizens, and will vote for whoever worked to get them the amnesty. The second thing I thought was, even though they are not on Medicaid, the American taxpayer is still paying for any and all the health care they receive.

NO PAYMENT IT'S FREE
All the laws that had been broken

As a home health care coordinator, I continued to see the cost of illegal immigration. I had to setup home health care for an illegal immigrant from Brazil who was injured working at a construction site. The scaffolding he was working on collapsed, and he broke both of his legs. The man was rushed to the hospital and underwent two operations to repair his legs. He spent thirty days total in the hospital receiving the best care the American medical system could provide. Now, I was to supply him with a walker, and bedside commode, and home physical therapy. While reviewing the chart I mentioned to the patient's doctor all the laws that had been broken. I said that "the man does not have a green card, so it's illegal to hire him, he does not have a social security number' so he is not paying income or social security tax." "His employer did not take workers comp. insurance out on him and that is illegal." Finally, I told the doctor "I will bet my life they are not paying him minimum wage." I also said to the doctor "the hospital will not receive any reimbursement for this man's care or for my services." The doctor responded that when he worked in Miami "this type of thing was common." I asked the doctor "how to hospitals survive in Miami. The doctor stated "federal aid." So again, we have some business people benefiting from illegal immigration and the American taxpayer is footing the bill.

IT'S ILLEGAL, BUT SO WHAT

While at work she died of a heart attack

In my thirty-eight years in nursing I have known four nurses who were narcotic abusers. Easy access to narcotics may be a reason for drug addiction among nurses. Nurses who are addicts will sign out narcotics for patients and never give them to the patient. Narcotics are usually written as P.R.N.s. That means the patient must ask for the drug. An example would be Percocet 1 every for hour for pain. If the patient is not in pain, he does not get the drug. I knew a male nurse who would sign out for pain pills and chart that they were given, and not administer them. If the patient was not in pain no one would be the wiser. The nurse was eventually caught and went through the impaired nurse's program, and eventually went back to work as an R.N. at another hospital. While at work he died from a heart attack related to his past abuse of drugs sitting in his truck in the hospital parking lot.

Another way nurses who are addicted obtain narcotics is by not giving patient the full dose of their medications. For example, if a patient has an order for morphine 4mg I.V. (intravenously) every 4 hours PRN, the nurse will give the parent 2mg and give herself 2mg. I knew an I.C.U. nurse who inserted an I.V. into her leg and was splitting I.V. pain medication between herself and the patient. She got caught because her job performance became substandard. She once tried to give an intramuscular injection using a blunt needle. Also, the oncoming shift noticed her patients were always in pain. Shortly after being discovered she died, I am not sure of the cause, but I can guess.

I worked at a small seventy bed hospital where they did

not lock up the Darvocet. Darvocet was a narcotic used in the treatment of mild to moderate pain (Darvocet is no longer on the market). After I was there for three years, the hospital hired an R.N. from up North. Within six months the pharmacy noticed on my floor, the Darvocet was missing. Hospital administration suspected the northern nurse because before she was employed, we never had a problem with missing drugs. They asked her for a urine sample, so they could run a drug screen. For some reason, the urine specimen was lost. After that, they started locking up the Darvocet and we treated it like all the other narcotics. This meant that a nurse from the off going shift, along with a nurse on coming shift, would have to count the drugs together and sign for them. One night she drew up Demerol in a syringe and went down the stairwell. When she came back on the floor the syringe was empty, and she tried to get another nurse to sign in the narcotics record book that she wasted the drug. The other nurse refused, saying that she did not witness the waste, and she called the nursing supervisor and informed her of the incident. The nursing supervisor sent the northern nurse home.This resulted in an investigation that revealed the northern nurse was not an R.N. The state she came from had reciprocity with Florida. That meant a nurse from Florida can work in that state under her Florida license, and a nurse from that northern state can work in Florida. It turned out the nurse was an L.P.N. What this L.P.N. did was copy the license number from an R.N. from her home state. She never showed human resources a license; instead she just gave them a license number. This resulted in the hospital being fined $10,000 for employing some one as an R.N. who did not have a R.N. license.

Not all nurses who become drug addicts obtain their narcotics from the hospital. I worked with a beautiful nurse who became a cocaine addict. She went on vacation with two other nurses and according to those nurses there was no end of guys who sought her attention. This nurse probably had an addictive personality. (they never do anything in moderation, it's all the way down on the gas, or all the way down on the brakes) She was a smoker and tried to give up cigarettes with the assistance of a nicotine patch. That was unsuccessful. In the morning you would see her coming to work, wearing the patch and smoking. (of course this gives her a double dose of nicotine) Three years after I met her, she married. Shortly after her marriage, someone introduced her to cocaine. Soon, she became addicted to cocaine. Within two years, she was divorced. While married she did have one child. For her drug addiction, she went through rehab three times. Her mother ended up raising her child. Due to her addiction she could not work as a nurse. By the time she was forty, she looked like she was sixty. She died shortly after her fortieth birthday. I never saw a drug addict in retirement.

BABIES

I described everything we saw to them

When I reported for work at this hospital, I was directed to the floor where infants and children were cared for. I got that assignment because no regular staff would float to that floor. (They were afraid to work there for reasons like, the medication doses were given through specialty pediatric equipment, and they couldn't start IV's on scared screaming fighting kids). I took anything they threw at me, it was all a day's work.

I arrived at the floor and was greeted by the only RN present who was regularly assigned to that area. She was glad to see me because there were always two nurses assigned there at all times. I took my direction from her, and was told to go into the nursery and check the babies and infants for diaper changes. There were three in there, and two were dirty, so I changed them and went for my next job.

The other nurse was giving attention to a little two year old boy that was shot by his father while cleaning his gun. The child's intestines were blown away and he was to have a colostomy bag for the rest of his life. The father was present caring for the tyke to give the mother time to go home and rest. The nurse told me that the court ordered him to care for the son until he was discharged, then he was to report to prison, he was already sentenced to several years for weapons offenses.

The three babies were all on IV medications because they were vaginal births and contracted diseases from their mothers at time of birth. The babies were all listed as "failure to thrive" because their mothers were prostitutes and wanted nothing to do with caring for their babies. Failure to thrive means that the babies have not bonded with their mothers, are not held and played with enough, and generally are listless from being ignored by the responsible parent. So, my job became getting the babies out of their bassinettes and dragging them around with me as I did every chore I could dream up. Including answering the phone calls. I would always have one or two with me all shift, we even took walks from one end of the unit to the other, while I described everything we saw to them. When they saw the two year old they were alert and very happy, and we followed the boy to the playroom where they watched him play with great interest. When they tired, I gave them a nap and grabbed another and away we went, they needed all the stimulation they could get. I felt so sorry for them knowing that they were not loved, but, I enjoyed making their day a happy one.

ANOTHER BABY STORY

It's almost impossible not to look at a baby

While operating an out-patient surgical center, I had every patient greeted at the door to the prep area when their name was announced. Of course, I took my turn greeting patients and welcoming them into the center. These times are very stressful for patients, and they welcome any kind of diversion that takes their mind off what is coming. I devised many "games" that we used to play with the patients, and one was reciting "Twas the night before Christmas." I would start by reciting the first verse, and point to the patient for the second verse, which they all knew. We would go on until the patient missed one (we knew the whole poem). We would give them the book with the poem to see, and when they were ready, we would do it again. One day every patient in the place wanted to play, and to our surprise, a patient who had been there a month before had gone home and memorized the poem hoping that we would play the game again, and we did. Everyone was amazed, and we and all the patients that day had a great laugh about it, we tried to make their visit anything but anxious.

On this day, I was retrieving a patient from the waiting room when I noticed a car seat on a chair with a baby in it. It is almost impossible not to go look at a baby when you spot their paraphernalia. Giving in to temptation, I went over to look at the baby, and what I saw drew me back in horror. There in the car seat was an infant all shriveled up like an old man. It didn't look like a baby at all, it looked like an infant ape. I asked the mother if the baby was ill, or trying to recover from an illness. She looked at me like I was nuts, and asked me why I asked that question. I retorted with the response that "babies don't look like that." She came back with "this baby is different, she is a vegan." I drew back in horror, now everything made horrible sense, the mother was starving the infant to death. A thousand things went through my mind in an instant, so many things that I was rendered speechless, and if you know me, that is virtually impossible. I turned and walked away, resolving to do something about this as fast as I could.

I quickly explained the problem to one of the female nurses, and asked her to go look at the baby in the waiting room. She went out, and asked to see the baby, and had the same reaction as I did. She sat down next to the mother and began to talk to her, which is what I wanted. She explained that being a vegan was a choice grown people make, but a baby is not a grown person who can make a choice like that. She explained that fats are needed by babies to assure normal growth and development, and her baby was devoid of any fat at all. Instead of being a big pink bundle, this infant was a wrinkled grey looking underweight skeleton. Finally, I asked one of the attending physicians to talk to the mother, and he agreed, but the mother took the baby out of the building to wait in her car for the patient she had driven to the center. I have often wondered if the baby survived, because I was sure the mother was set in her ways and wouldn't listen to common sense. It's the same old story, you can't talk rationally to irrational people.

IS ALCOHOL IS A DRUG?
She had been drinking wine all morning

When you are appointed to run or control an organization, lots of thing can go wrong, and do. But it is never fun when something happens that has the potential to ruin everything. This story highlights the issue that there is no set way to tackle the unforeseen actions of a wayward employee. Or, several wayward employees at almost the same time, it's a nightmare.

An outpatient surgical center has a unique set of rules very similar to a hospital, but everything happening there must conclude at the close of business every day. There are numerous drugs in the building which are under double lock, and stay under double lock 24 hours a day. A pharmacist stocks the drug supply and the nurses draw from it and sign for everything needed on orders from the doctor. Every evening a cleaning crew comes to the center after hours and cleans the patient care areas, with the exception of the hallway leading to the procedure rooms, and the procedure rooms. I would not let them enter the area where the procedures were done, only the RN's entered or cleaned these areas. The medications, however were kept in a separate locked room close to the patient care area, and behind the reception area.

One morning an RN went to get a medication from the med room, and noticed that two vials of valium were missing from the last pack in the pile of valium supplies. This was unusual, because we always issued them in order starting from the top to the bottom. Someone had manipulated the supply and illegally stole two vials. I immediately suspected the cleaning crew, so I reported the loss through channels and a drug screen was ordered on all of the employees and the cleaning crew. The screen consisted of cutting a few strands of everyone's hair for testing. If a substance was found in the hair, the employee had the burden of producing a prescription for that drug. If they could not produce a script, then appropriate action would be taken.

All of the nurses cleared the drug screen, the 2nd girl in reception showed cannabis, and the cleaning crew refused to show for the testing at their appointed time. I called the cleaning company and informed them that the cleaning company was fired for refusing their drug tests. The 2nd girl in reception was also replaced because we had to have a drug free environment. And this was the start of my problems with employees in the surgical center.

About a week later after everything had settled down, I was in the drug room getting a medication for a procedure when a doctor entered the room to talk to me in private. I had been working in a procedure room all day, and this was just after lunch when she approached me. She reported that one of the nurses was possibly intoxicated and she did not want that nurse to be in touch with any of her patients. I was shocked to say the least, so I gave the meds to another RN to take them to the procedure room, and asked the RN working with the suspect nurse if she had noticed anything strange going on. She reported that the nurse had come back from lunch intoxicated, or at least it appeared that way. I immediately accosted her, and told her to stop work and leave the building, she was through for the day. We finished the day and I gathered the other nurses together, and asked them if they had ever seen this type of behavior from her before, and they all said yes. I had not noticed anything because I usually worked in the procedure rooms because the girls hated wearing lead garments during procedures. I decided to wait until the next morning to see the nurse privately, face to face about her issue.

The next day the nurse did not show up for work in the AM. About 10 O'clock I received a phone call from her, and she was drunk. Most of what she said was unintelligible, but I got the idea that she was concerned about being fired from the job. She told me that she was drinking wine all morning, and was thinking about getting help with her drinking. I heard nothing for several days, calling in one of my part time RN's to fill her slot. Finally, after three days I received a call from her husband telling me that she was in a rehab facility. He asked for a guarantee that I would hold her job for her, which I denied. I told him she could reapply when she straightened out, and her full time RN position would be filled immediately because the work load dictated full staffing. He was not happy with my answer. I also suspected that she had been dismissed from her prior job working in a hospital based out-patient surgical center. Those jobs were plum jobs in a hospital, and no one quits a plum job like that. She never got her job back, but sued me privately for dismissing her, because of extreme prejudice against her. The suit went nowhere because she had to pay out of her pocket to keep it going, and I was defended by the lawyers for the surgical center. After the initial paperwork on the case, I never saw anything else from her.

Several years later when I was teaching a clinical nursing class in the open-heart unit of a hospital, she was admitted in critical condition with an overdose and survived, that was the last time I ever saw her. I was aware that she had lost her RN license, or surrendered it, because she was missing from the RN database. Since writing this story I found out she died in 2017.

BLACK BLOOD

In a few minutes he came out to see me
and he was pale as a ghost

I had an assignment to visit an elderly man who lived in a small first floor unit in a group of apartments. I enjoyed seeing him because he was such a friendly fellow. He was beset with problems related to diabetes and circulation which tended to get out of hand, probably related to his diet. He was a widower with very limited funds, so his diet suffered as a result of his inability to purchase high quality food. I used to see him on a Monday morning at about 9 o'clock in the morning. He always offered me a cup of coffee every time I visited, but I made it a practice of never accepting anything offered by patients, plus I hated the taste of coffee anyway. This was going to be a case of never ending visits because I saw no prospect of him changing anything around, or acquiring more finances, he was just making the rent payments, and his furniture was cast-offs.

I had been seeing him for about a month, and the visits were routine, with vital signs, a short assessment, and a question and answer period which he enjoyed immensely. I knew that he had no social life, and he waited every Monday for someone to talk to who was flesh and blood, like so many of my elderly patients living alone. They tended to sit by the window the day of my visit in anticipation of my arrival, and this guy was no different. He always had a topic to discuss which centered around what I was doing, and where and how I lived, he wanted to know everything. He seemed to take pleasure on me doing well, and took great interest in knowing that I was making great choices in life.

On this particular morning, he was not at the window

waiting for me. I immediately suspected that something was wrong. It was a Monday morning, so I had not seen him all weekend. He was not in the small living room area, he was in the bathroom. In a few minutes he came out to see me and he was pale as a ghost. He looked like he did not have an ounce of blood left in his body, he was wet looking and appeared dizzy and very frail. I had him sit down in a chair, and went to work getting a set of vital signs. I was struck by the fact that he had virtually no blood pressure. He told me that he noticed something wrong Friday night when he had a bout of diarrhea. He said that the stool was a blackish color, and it made him feel weak afterwards. He said that the diarrhea continued through the weekend, even at night. I went to the bathroom and looked at the toilet, and the sides of the bowl was covered with digested blood, black as pitch. This was a symptom of a stomach ulcer, because the blood was not red, but digested by the system. (remember, blood has protein in it) I dialed 911 and admonished the man because he should have called over the weekend himself. He said he was looking forward to my visit on Monday and he knew that I would "get him fixed up."

Off he went to the ER and three pints of packed red cells, and a stomach lavage to clot off the bleeder which was caused by his medications being taken without adequate food or fluids. Medications for the most part are acids, or salts, so adequate food must be taken with most medications, even an aspirin tablet which is acetylsalicylic ACID.

BOY ARE YOU IN TROUBLE

It was necessary to remove all of the intestines

A patient came into the emergency room with severe chest pain. After examination and careful study of his test results and scans, he was diagnosed with a dissecting aortic aneurysm. This is a problem most associated with higher blood pressures. The high pressures cause blisters in the arterial wall which cause tears in the lining of the blood vessel. Blood under high pressure courses into the tear and rips a separation between the linings of the blood vessel. (the best example of this is when you are putting on a winter coat and your arm goes through a tear in the coat sleeve lining, and your arm slides down between the lining and the sleeve trapping your arm inside the sleeve)

The condition becomes fatal if it is not treated quickly, and in this case a surgeon was chosen from the ER list and the OR was prepped for surgery. The operation is not frequently done because it is not a common condition. The patient had the unlucky prospect of having the absolutely worst surgeon on the list be selected for the operation, simply because it was his turn at bat on the list. Not knowing this the patient was taken to the OR and the surgery was attempted. In this case the section of the aorta was being replaced with a graft. It was necessary to remove all of the intestines to work on the graft. The intestines, still connected, were laid on the OR table until the surgery was completed, then they were replaced into the body and the wound was sutured shut. The operation is extensive, although if well done it is a total cure for the problem.

Post surgery, the patient was admitted to the surgical ICU unit for recovery. Everyone employed at the hospital was waiting to see how the patient was going to progress, because this doctor had a long history of either having to redo surgeries, or botching them up where they could not be fixed. It was with baited breath that we all waited for daily reports on the patient through the hospital grapevine. Several days post-op the patient sat up in bed, and had his first light meal, he was fine. It didn't seem like a miracle, it was a miracle.

I happened upon the surgeon in the elevator a week later, and congratulated him on the successful aortic surgery. He said "it was one of those cases where everything just fell into place so easily, I just knew it was going to be a good outcome" He was right, the patient was fixed and the discharge was uneventful. This proves the old saying, "even a blind squirrel finds a nut once in a while."

BRAIN INJURY
I had been set-up by the female nurses

I reported to the nursing office for my assignment, and I was sent to a lockdown unit for brain damaged patients. These units are meant to contain patients that may be mobile, but do not have cognitive thought. (they can't think like you and me) They are prone to wandering, and locking down the unit assures everyone that they stay within prescribed boundaries. Brain damaged patients fall within certain groups, the largest of which are motorcycle riders. Almost half of the patients were drunk driving motorcycles at night, and had one vehicle accidents. (only the motorcycle was involved) They usually were going fast and misjudged a curve and ran off the road and crashed. Very few were wearing helmets, and those that were received closed head brain injuries. All of them in the unit had received severe brain injuries, and were alive in body only.

In one particular case a young man about thirty had a very pleasant wife, and a new baby, who came to spend time with him almost every day. The nurses on the unit explained that the wife had been beaten by the husband in drunken rages while she was pregnant. The husband was described as a "bad actor." This guy required complete care which was feeding, washing, changing, everything you could think of. His discharge was looming, and the doctor wanted to make arrangements for his placement in a facility. (there are human warehouses where patients are placed permanently until death) The wife objected, and wanted the patient sent home with her and the baby. She said she would provide all the care necessary for his well-being. Therefore, she was trained by the nurses in preparation for discharge. The feeling was that she was going to get even with the bastard for all the beatings she got from him. I'm willing to bet that what the nurses thought was the truth.

The second type of patients in the unit, were falls, where the patient struck their head really hard. This type of patient usually had a physical disability from the fall, and a closed head brain injury too. Unbelievably, most of these injuries were the do-it-yourself husbands, who always said "I'll just throw a ladder up, and do it myself it will only take a minute." There were more of this type than one would realize, I certainly didn't. They were usually not as bad as the motorcycle group, and could be led around like they were in a daze, and some would even follow simple instruction like "sit down."

The third type were a mix of automobile accident, bar fights, roofers, and bicycle rider-car collisions, but they were by far in the minority. One of the most notable cases in this group was a young woman in her twenties who was in a terrible car accident in Nevada. Both her and a friend were travelling at night on one of those highways with no speed limit when the accident occurred. Everyone involved in the accident was killed at the scene but her, and she was mangled in the wreckage and had to be extricated. From the looks of her, you would think she was at fault, because she at twenty something, was covered with grotesque tattoos. After seeing her, two things came to mind, a motorcycle gang, or a rock star groupie.

Nurses like to play sick jokes on each other when possible, so me being agency I was not familiar with this female patient. The staff nurses knew that this female had no inhibitions and would immediately offer me all kinds of sexual favors through her slurred speech. They were watching and waiting for me to get into the room to pass my meds and see if she needed any care that I would provide. As I made my rounds, they were watching me like a hawk when I entered her room. I approached the bed and the patient asked me if I had come to "get some." Me being a dumb ass, asked her "get some of what"? She flung back her covers revealing that she had pulled her gown up and was showing me her vagina. I heard a lot of giggling at that point and realized that I had been set up by the female nurses watching from around the doorway. They all knew what was going to happen with that patient. The worst part of the whole thing was I had a tough time all night wrestling with her trying to keep her from grabbing me in the wrong places, she was a trip. I was glad when that night was over, and although I was assigned there numerous times, I never had her again.

THE ROOFER
I might make the pond

This group of stories brings to mind the story of a roofer who avoided the brain injury route by some quick thinking and manual dexterity. The roofer was working three stories up, on a shingle roof. He told me that there were strips of wood nailed to the bottom of the roof to prevent falling off. If you slid down the slope of the roof, your feet would catch the strip and stop the slide before you went over the edge. He had finished a section, and was walking along the roof to a new spot when he stepped on a loose shingle laying on top of the ones nailed down. The shingle slid and he went with it, falling onto the roof. He began to slide down the roof feet first, when to his horror he saw that there was no strip of wood there to stop his slide. His mind raced for the several seconds his slide took. He was trying to picture what was below the roof at that section of the property. He remembered a concrete walkway directly below, a small section of grass lawn, and a retention pond after the grass. As he slid, he thought that if he could hit the ground at the retention pond, he might survive the fall. When he reached the edge of the roof feet first, he pushed off as hard as he could from the edge of the roof with both hands hoping it would propel him the distance to the pond. When he pushed off hard, it had the effect of turning him over so his feet faced the building, and his head out toward the pond, he thought that this was a good, though unexpected thing. With his back toward the ground and his face toward the sky, he made his descent. He tried to look down as he saw that he had already passed the concrete walkway, and was over the grass plot. As the fall continued, he thought "I might make the pond" as he crashed to the ground halfway into the pond and halfway onto the lawn and tall grass at the end of the pond. His head splashed into the 10 in. deep water and soft muck in the pond, and he immediately knew he would be OK. He suffered a back injury and leg injuries, but he recovered and avoided the brain injury unit altogether.

CAN I STILL USE COCAINE
I told him to stop taking drugs

Drug addiction is a terrible monkey to have on your back. I have seen forty year old drug addicts who looked like they were sixty. I thank God I never developed that vice. Unlike T.V. where drug addicts tend to be people of color and ghetto dwellers, many addicts are white and middle class. In the 1980s, cocaine was the drug of choice among the white middle and upper classes. One such patient showed up in our E.R. He was a thirty-one year old salesman who was complaining of chest pain. An E.K.G. was done and it showed him to be in tachycardia (a heart beat greater than 100 beats a minute) with frequent P.V.C.s (premature ventricle contractions). This condition is something you do not expect to find in a thirty-one year old male. He admitted to the E.R. doctor that he was a cocaine user.

He was transferred to the telemetry unit for heart monitoring. While sitting at the desk watching the heart monitor (the monitor tech was at lunch) this man approached me and wanted to know how his heart was doing. I told him not well. His heart beat was rapid with frequent P.V.C.s. This means his heart was not efficiently working. He asked me what he could do about this. I asked him if he was doing drugs. He replied yes he was using cocaine and marijuana. I told him to stop taking drugs. He left and went back to his room. Five minutes later he returned and asked me if he stopped using marijuana could he still use cocaine. I told him no, he looked disappointed and returned to his room.

I do not know what happened to this man. I had the next two days off. When I returned to work he was discharged. My guess is he did not have a long life. Despite fearing for his life, he still did not want to give up cocaine. Today I see am seeing more white middle class drug addicts, this time the drug of choice is Oxycontin. In fact, one of the hospitals I worked at had an entire thirty-eight bed unit filled with Oxycontin addicts.

20% of cocaine addicts take it to the grave, 80 % of cigarette smokers take it to the grave. The man had an 80% chance that he would quit before he was killed by the addiction, of course, unless he was an idiot.

CHARGE NURSE OOPS

I decided to go back to the room and stay there

Some patients need temporary dialysis especially when they are so sick their kidneys can't filter the blood anymore. In these cases, large IV and arterial lines are started on the side of the neck. These lines are used by the dialysis nurse to connect the patient to the dialysis machine. (The machine filters the blood by exposing it to a sterile fluid where the exchange of waste products takes place)

The patient in this story was at dialysis when I started the shift. Halfway through the shift he came rolling up the hallway in a wheelchair pushed by the dialysis nurse. We got him settled in his room, and I went about my normal work. The patient was about 40 years old and in reasonable physical shape. Approximately fifteen minutes later, the dialysis patients light came on and I went to the room to check on him. He reported a funny feeling in his neck, so, I looked closely, but could see nothing apparent, however he seemed really concerned about it.

I went to the charge nurse a prior CCU nurse, and asked him to take a look at the patient. He walked up to the room, and examined the patient also. He reported to me that the patient seemed nervous, and to give him a valium for anxiety. I had seen patients acting like this in the past, and I felt that something was wrong with the lines used by the dialysis nurse. I seemed pretty sure that one of the lines was leaking blood into the neck even though nothing was visible to the eye. I decided to go back to the room and stay there to make sure that the patient would get help if he needed it. When I walked into the room the patient was out of bed standing between the bed and the wall in a small space. He seemed really upset this time and grabbed me by both arms. He started coughing trying to clear his throat, but was unsuccessful, even though I could hear him inhaling and exhaling lots of air. At that time, I was sure that this patient was going to code. I tried to get past him to mash the code button on the wall, but he was blocking my path and holding onto me by both my arms. I could see that he was so worked up that he was putting an oxygen demand on his system that it could not furnish. I knew there was no sense in me wrestling with the patient to get past him to the code button. I could see that he was on the verge of falling into unconsciousness, so I just waited a few more seconds and true to my prediction he passed out. I caught him on the way down and managed to toss him onto his bed and mash the code button at the same time.

I began positioning the bed and patient for the code team a few of which started to stream through the door of the room. I explained the patient's complaint about his neck, and related my thoughts about the dialysis nurse dislodging one of the lines in his neck during the procedure. He had a tube passed into his airway just in time, because the blood in his neck was pushing the trachea to the side and it was becoming almost impossible to access it. Once the clear airway was established and the patient oxygenated, he was out of immediate danger. Unfortunately, I had to call the code team to get the tube placed in his airway, there was no way for a floor nurse to accomplish that in the room. He was removed to CT scan and then moved to the surgical intensive care unit.

Four months later I was working on the floor in the hall preparing medications to be given when a man approached me. He looked familiar, but when he began to speak, I recognized him as the fellow I had coded. He said "I want to thank you for saving my life", he had remembered me. I told him he had such a grip on me I couldn't do anything until he went unconscious. He related to me that when all was said and done, that I was right all along, and what I thought was wrong, was exactly what it turned out to be. He had pulled through everything, and did not need dialysis any more, he looked the picture of health. He was the only patient in 18 years who ever said thanks.

WAS IT FUN IN THE SUN?

The boy saw this as an opportunity to jump the wake

Working the evening shift at a trauma center, I was assigned a patient that had been airlifted to the hospital and placed on my unit while the operating room was being prepped. I was required to do frequent vital signs on her according to a pre-planned routine. The 20+ year old girl was shaking like a leaf from both pain and from being scared for her future, post incident. Her parents were at the bedside as well as her boyfriend who was with her at the time of the accident. As I took the vital signs, she was trying to explain what had transpired during a fun day out with her boyfriend.

Both the boyfriend and the patient had decided it would be fun to go to a local oceanside hotel and rent a jet ski. There are a few hotels that have a line stretched between the beach and a small raft placed out in the water maybe 50 ft. away. Tethered alongside the rope are jet skis and sitting on the raft are additional jet skis all ready for rental. A sea doo jet ski is essentially a motorcycle that travels on water. Most young people do not consider that a jet ski can be dangerous. They look on it as a big toy to go out and play on in the water. They feel that you can't get hurt because all that can happen is you will fall off into the water, and that is better than crashing a motorcycle onto the road. The jet skis have a lanyard attached to the driver to shut off the motor if the driver should fall off the ski.

The young couple were out having fun spinning the jet ski in circles, and jumping wakes almost always at full throttle. The ski is propelled by a column of water being ejected out the back of the ski under tremendous pressure giving it the thrust to obtain lots of speed quickly. There is no danger of being struck by a propeller and sliced to pieces. The young woman was sitting behind the driver straddling the seat with her feet in the trough on each side of the ski. A large boat went by the couple, and the boy saw this as an opportunity to jump the wake and possibly "get a little air." He went full blast toward the wake and hit the first wave head on. The small craft did fly up almost vertical and the girl lost her grip and slid back on the seat and fell off the ski with her legs spread wide apart. She dropped directly into the path of the jet stream of water coming out the nozzle from the powerful jacuzzi pump. The column of water sliced through her flimsy bikini bottom and continued to slice its way into her vagina. It sliced through her vagina, destroyed the tissue separating her anus from the vagina, and continued to slice into her internal organs giving her a massive wound between her legs. It was no wonder she was shaking so bad, given the trauma she had experienced. The hospital was waiting for both a reconstructive surgeon and a gynecologist to come in from home to take the patient to surgery.

The girl was eventually taken to the OR and remained there through my shift, I never saw her again. Who would think that a ride on a jet ski would lead to life changing injuries.

THE BRAIN IS FRAGILE
He was big into motorcycles

I received a transfer from the ICU of a man who had been in a coma since admission. He was the victim of an accident between an automobile and a motorcycle. In his accident, he was broadsided by the automobile emerging from a day care parking lot onto a main road. The driver of the car a female reported that she did not see the motorcycle because she was texting her husband, telling him that she had picked up the daughter from daycare. The impact crushed the left leg of the motorcycle operator and flung him to the road mashing his helmet in the process. In addition to multiple fractures to the leg, he suffered a closed head injury causing a coma.

The rider was married with no children, and his wife and family visited daily, sitting by the bedside. The attending neurologist had explained to the family that it was very possible that the patient would not wake up, and if he did not, he wouldn't last long in this condition. At the bedside the family discussed which funeral director they were going to use, and what clothing he would wear, etc. They were making plans based on the doctor's diagnosis, which they had come to believe was the only option. The patient was a pretty big fellow, and aside from the leg, looked the picture of good health. I had been taking care of him for almost a week, and his vital signs were very stable. I had been moving him side to side to prevent bed sores which you do 24 hours a day.

One night, I was roughing him up trying to get him in a good position laying on his side, by stuffing pillows under him to hold him in position. All of a sudden, he said "what the hell is going on" I was stunned, he had awakened from his coma, and was somewhat lucid. I walked around the bed, and looked into his face, and his eyes were open. I told him that he was in the hospital, and I was his nurse. He said "a man nurse, what is the chance I would get a man nurse." I explained that I was the only one on the floor big enough to muscle him around, and he laughed. I told him I was leaving the room to call his doctor, and I would be back.

When I returned, he began to relate a story to me about the accident he was involved in. He was big into motorcycles, and was coming from a parts store where he had bought some chrome pieces to put on his bike. After a few blocks he got stuck in traffic because of an accident a block away. When he got up to the accident, he saw the victim lying on the roadway dead, and the motorcycle was crushed. Fifteen blocks further, he was stuck in traffic again because of another motorcycle accident, and again, he saw the body on the road flailing around from injuries. He was scared out of his wits, and resolved that he would sell the bike when he got home, and quit riding motorcycles. Two blocks from home he was struck and almost killed, and he reported that somehow, he knew that everything would be all right because he had a feeling of serenity immediately after the impact.

The family was notified, and came to the hospital right away to see him. He was very calm with them as if only one day had passed since he saw them, and it had been almost 5 days. He told them that after his leg was healed, he never wanted to ride another motorcycle again. He wanted to buy a big 4 wheel drive truck because he didn't want to go through this again.

SOMETHING I DIDN'T KNOW
Everyone running into one of my rooms

When a patient is admitted by a physician to a hospital, of course the family doctor knows everything about the patient, and writes the orders to be followed concerning patient care. In the following case everything had been done long before I had come to work on that floor of the hospital. I received report from the RN leaving the floor which included basic information like vital signs, diet, and any ongoing problems that needed to be addressed during my shift. When a patient has been on the floor for several days, they are usually accommodated to the hospital workings and become less and less needy. That was the case with every patient that I was assigned to take care of on this particular day, they had all been there for three days or more, so I was looking forward to a routine shift.

On day shift, both meds and meals tend to overlap which is not a bad thing because most medications are either salts or acids, and they go better with food than just a glass of water. That is why prescription meds at home have a label on the container saying take with food.

I went in to each patients room and looked them over while I did vital signs, and they were all awake and sitting up awaiting breakfast. While in the room I move the over the bed table into position and cleared a space on it to receive the food tray. You have to accomplish multiple tasks while you are in each room to eliminate running back and forth all day because you were stupid and forgot something you had to do, it's called working smart. I took no particular notice of anything while moving from room to room, everything seemed completely normal when the trays arrived on the floor. It is the nurse's job to pass each and every tray for their assigned patients. I went to the cart and matched the dietary slips on the cart to my printed notes on diet for each patient, and began passing out the trays. After I would finish the trays, I would do the med pass while the patients had the food and drink in front of them. I reached the room across from the nurses station and entered with the first tray which was for the patient near the window of the room. This gentleman had his wife with him in the cubicle, and she took possession of the tray and began to prepare it for her husband. The curtain was drawn between the beds so the patients had privacy. I went out and retrieved the tray for the patient next to the door and placed it on the bedside table and asked the patient if he needed help with the tray, and he indicated no by moving his head. Before I left the room, he had picked up a muffin on the tray and bit into it dropping lots of crumbs in the process. I readjusted the tray to catch any other droppings, and instructed him to take his time with the meal there was no hurry to eat it quickly. I had the med cart in front of the next room so I began to prepare medications for that group of patients first. I had just finished putting the first meds into the plastic cup when I noticed panic at the charge nurse desk and everyone running into one of my rooms. The wife of the patient in the window bed had gone to the nurses station outside the room and reported that she thought she heard the patient choking. I turned and also ran to the room and witnessed my patient choking on scrambled eggs. We went to work on hm first by trying to clear his mouth and trying the Heimlich maneuver on him. A code was called immediately, and the code team arrived and began working on him. We assisted as needed, but in a short time the code was called off and the patient was pronounced dead. After the death I rechecked the diet and saw that all was as it should be, but I could not understand why the patient all of a sudden had trouble with food, or swallowing the food. The charge nurse received a call from the police department and the officer on the phone asked to speak to me. The charge nurse refused to put me on the phone, telling the officer "you do whatever you have to do, and I'll do whatever I have to do, but you are not talking to the assigned nurse." The officer hung up and we all went about our normal routine and nothing more was said that day.

The next day I was to work the same unit on the same shift with all the same staff. The charge nurse had received information when she took report that there were big problems associated with the death of the patient the day before. The story goes as follows:

The patient was admitted through the ER and a physician was assigned from a list kept in the ER. In this case, the assigned doctor did not know the patient prior to the admission. Basic orders were written for the patient which included a diet. However, before the patient received a tray, he had a med pass and the nurse gave him the meds and a glass of water to take them with. The patient had problems drinking and taking the meds (which is done in front of the nurse to be sure the meds are taken) he choked all over the place, so the nurse cancelled the diet and made a call asking the covering physician for a swallow study. This was three days before the patient died. The swallow study was performed, and the patient was ordered to be NPO which means nothing by mouth. (a swallow study is conducted by a nurse, or a dietitian using liquids of various consistency, from very thick to thin like water, the liquids are fed to the patient using a spoon, and the ability of the patient to control the liquids is noted) An IV was hung and the patient was given fluids continuously. The patient continued NPO for the next two days because the assigned physician took no action on the swallow study.

Late in the afternoon the day before my shift, the assigned doctor visited the patient saw the IV bag hanging and discontinued the IV in preparation for discharge the next morning. What he did not do was find the swallow study ordered previously by the covering physician. Not seeing the study, he put the patient on a regular diet, which was reported to me by the night shift nurse. The patient was going to be discharged sometime after breakfast to a group home where he lived, he was mentally retarded which was never reported to me either. The swallow study was two days old and back several pages in the chart. When I received report, the diet was a regular diet so there was no indication that a problem would surface on my shift. The doctor was questioned extensively, and was really caught with his pants down, but nothing was done to him. At a later date I was questioned by a department of health death investigator, but I had broken no protocols so it was just a formality.

THE HAIRDRESSER

"Here we go again with the neighbor helping story"

Alone, a dilapidated house, unable to clean themselves, virtually unable to make food, underweight, chronic debilitating ailments, and no common sense. This is the conditions that many elderly people live under every day, and this is one such story of leading a horse to water, pushing their head down into the water, and still they won't drink. (a metaphor)

I was agency and was assigned to cover a home health RN who was on vacation. My duties were to drive to each patient's home and treat according to the treatment plan left at the patient's residence. Everything was going along swimmingly until I got to an old frame single home in a row of post war bungalow's built for returning soldiers after WW 2. I knocked at the front door, and thirty flakes of old paint fell off the door and hit the ground in front of me. I heard a faint "come in" obviously a very old person was speaking from inside. I walked into the small living room, and saw no one obviously present in the front room or small kitchen. The house reeked of stale air and unwashed flesh, an "old lady" smell. I called out "hello" and heard a small voice say "I'm back here, come on back." Right away, I knew this was going to be a nightmare case. I walked into the bedroom off the kitchen, and lying in a bed in the room was an aged relic of a time long past. The very elderly woman was still in bed with the covers pulled all the way up to her chin. The bed had not been changed in months, or possibly years, it stunk. I set to work getting her vital signs, and pulled the chart open to review her needs. I saw that she had one week of visits because of a change in her medications that the doctor thought might compromise her blood pressure.

Today was the last visit, and I was sent to sign off of the case. Since this visit was after one o'clock PM I inquired why she was still in bed. She informed me that when she rolled over that night she was struck with a terrible pain in her back, and could not rise up from the bed because of severe pain. I knew immediately what her problem was, she had Osteoporosis and had broken a vertebra when she twisted to roll over. I informed her of the probable cause of her back pain and reported that I was going to call 911 and send her to the emergency room. She immediately rebelled, and said she would refuse to leave her house. Of course, that created a dilemma, because the fire rescue would not take a person who refused service. I called her physician and was instructed to send her to the ER, and after she talked to her own doctor, she again refused service. I went to the kitchen and looked in the refrigerator, and there was only a small amount of left overs in there to eat, nothing else. I asked her how she was going to live in the bed for the weeks it would take to enable her to function again, and she said she would manage with the help of neighbors next door. "here we go again with the neighbor helping story I had heard so many times before" To me it sounded like "the dog ate my homework."

At this point let's do a little background info on this patient to help you understand how she wound-up in this predicament. She was one of three children of her parents, one boy and two girls. She was the baby, consequently, she was spoiled rotten by her parents. The boy, making his way in the world, went to school and became a doctor, and was drafted into the army after medical school. The sister also went to school and became a registered nurse, and the baby became a hairdresser. There were problems between siblings as there are in some families, and they sometimes fought over things. One day when her brother was visiting from a military base nearby, she got into a very heated argument with her brother, and was struck in the face, giving her a black eye. She was pissed, so she got dressed up in her finest and with a pair of dark sunglasses went to the base to seek out her brother's commanding officer. She found him without too much problem (because she was a very good looking blonde) and saw him in his office. She explained that her brother had struck her in an argument, and showed the commanding officer her black eye when she removed her glasses. The commanding officer had a shit fit, he told her that he would personally see to the brother's discipline.

She was informed by letter several days later that the brother forfeited six month's pay, and was confined to barracks for six months after duty hours. That meant that he could not visit the family for six months. Furthermore, if he made contact with his sister again, he would be subject to a court's martial, and receive a dishonorable discharge, because he was already slapped with a Conduct Unbecoming an Officer.

She went on as a hairdresser and when her sister's husband died later in life, she moved in with her sister. Since she had been a hairdresser all her life, and had made good money she had lived very good. She had never married, but had loads of fun, but banked almost nothing, and had no pension plan for old age. Her sister supported her, for the most part, and when the sister died, she inherited the home they occupied. She collected welfare and her care was provided by Medicaid.

Back to the story, I went next door, and inquired of the helping neighbors, who stated that they didn't know her. Since she was to be discharged, I put a hold on it, and when I returned to the office, I told the case manager about the refusal to seek treatment, and left it in her hands. It was impossible for the patient to remain in her home, and possibly she needed a day or two to let it sink into her head that her refusal was stupid. She was afraid that going to the hospital would lead to an admission to a nursing home, and no old people want to go to a nursing home.

SAD CASES

These cases are all beyond the scope of modern medicine

Modern medicine can only do so much for a patient. The best nursing care can help heal bodies, but it cannot in these cases restore a person to who they were before. Working as a nurse you see a lot of sad cases that are emotionally stressful. Here are a few that come to mind. The first story happened in the mid-80s. When the A.I.D.S. epidemic first came on the scene, blood was not tested for the virus. As a result, many innocent people became infected and died from A.I.D.S. I took care of one of these innocent people. The patient in question was a sixty year old male who was married, had three children, and two grandchildren. Two years before, he had an operation at the same hospital where he became an A.I.D.S. patient. We were 99% sure he got the disease from blood he received in the hospital. Shortly after he was diagnosed, he died. He was a man who should have lived another twenty years. He should have seen his grandchildren get married. He should have enjoyed retirement with his wife, but instead through no fault of his own he was dead. When he died, I remember looking at his wife. She had the same look in her eyes (the thousand mile stare) that you see on soldiers suffering from combat fatigue.

It is always sad to see someone die before their time. I had a fifty nine year old woman who was diagnosed with end stage renal disease. This meant, for the rest of her life, she would have to report to a dialysis center three times a week. Usually the dialysis treatments at the center would last three to four hours. She did not want to live her life like that, so she went to the tub room for a bath, and twenty minutes later she was found dead. She filled up the bath tub with warm water then pulled out her dialysis shunt. When her nurse went to check on her, she was dead. She bled to death.

Finally, I had to care for a beautiful nineteen year old girl, who suffered traumatic brain injury. While texting and driving her car, she ran into the back of a bus, which left her with a brain injury. As a result of her brain injury, she could not feed herself. A tube had to be placed through her abdomen into her stomach (P.E.G. tube). For the rest of her life, she would be on tube feedings. The P.E.G. tube was hooked to a feeding pump that infused liquid formula that looked like a milk shake into her stomach. This is how she would receive nutrition for the rest of her life. Due to urinary incontinence, she had a urinary catheter inserted in her bladder. This is also something she would need for the rest of her life and would leave her prone to urinary tract infections. A hospital bed was delivered to her parents' house. Once she left the hospital her parents were responsible for her care, which included turning her every two hours to ensure she did not get bed sores. The only help the family would receive was a home health care nurse who would come by once a week and a home health care aide who would come by three times a week to assist in her bath. Instead of being in a hospital bed, this beautiful girl should have been going to parties and dating. I wonder what was so important that she could not pull off the road to send a message

One of the saddest cases I have seen was that of a twenty-eight year old man who was severely beaten by a group of bikers. This man was in the process of getting a divorce from his wife. The wife had run off and joined a biker gang. For some reason she had a falling out with the gang, so she fled to her estranged husband for safety. Gang members showed up at her husband's house, and while husband was protecting his wife, they gave him a beating. I felt it was odd that she did not have a mark on her. After the bikers left, she managed to get him into a car and drive him to the E.R., where she told the doctor his injuries were the result of a fall. The E.R. physician did not believe her and called the police.

As far as I know, she refused to name the assailants and no arrests were made, the husband was in no condition to talk.

The husband was moved to the neurology intensive care unit. He spent three months on that unit before he was moved to the neurology floor. He spent nine months on the neurology floor, where he received physical, occupational therapy and speech therapy. After nine months, he could walk with a walker and feed himself if someone setup his meal tray. He still had difficulty speaking. His difficulty with speech caused him a great deal of frustration, he also drooled a lot. While he was on the neurology floor, we think the gang made an attempt on his life. When the night nurse was making her rounds, well after visiting hours were over, she entered his room and found a man standing over his bed. Upon being discovered, the man fled almost knocking over the nurse. His wife only visited him twice when he was in intensive care, and never when he was moved to the floor.

After one year in the hospital, he was moved to the rehab center. As a result of his hospitalization, he lost all his possessions. (house, car and clothes).   Before he was transferred to rehab the nurses chipped in and bought him, underwear, socks, shoes, and couple of shirts and a couple of pairs of pants. I do not know what happened to him after he was moved to rehab. I have no idea if he was ever again able to live on his own or hold a job.

I worked part-time for two years for a nursing agency. They would send me to a hospital that was a trauma center in the southern part of my county. Usually I worked on their telemetry unit, but once I worked in their neurology intensive care unit. My patient that day was a twenty-one year old white male who suffered traumatic brain injury. When his mother visited, I learned what had happened. According to his mother, the patient lived at home with his mother and grandmother. After visiting a local bar, he came home and spoke briefly to his mother before going to bed. His mother said nothing seemed wrong at the time. When he failed to wake up for breakfast his grandmother tried to wake him. She was unable to arouse him, so she called the mother. The mother noticed blood on his pillow where his head lay and was unable to wake him, so she called 9/11. Besides a wound in the back of the head, the paramedics discovered bruises on his body. The sheriff's department was then called.

Since the county they lived in did not have a hospital with a trauma center he was flown by helicopter to the hospital where I worked though the agency. The patient had been in the neurology unit two weeks by the time I was caring for him. He had a feeding tube inserted through his nose into his stomach. He also had a Foley Catheter inserted into his bladder for elimination of urine. He did not respond to verbal or physical stimuli. Everyday, his mother made a sixty mile trip to the hospital to visit her son. She told me the sheriff's department theorized that her son heard a noise in the night and went to investigate it, and was attacked. No arrests were made in the case. A more likely scenario was a bar fight which left him with the head wound which was concealed by his hair, which he did not tell his mother about when he arrived home. Going to bed would give the subdural hematoma (blood clot on the brain) time to form and enlarge. After that shift I never saw the patient again, so I did not know what his final outcome was, but I know it wasn't good.

I had taken care of another patient with traumatic brain injury two times. This young man was a graduate from a local high school. He was a good looking boy from a nice family. He received a football scholarship to a college in another state. While at college he went to a party. At the party, he was attacked by a group of gang bangers. The gang members gave him a horrendous beating from which he never recovered.

Today, he lives at home with his family. He is fed through a tube inserted in his stomach. He has a trachea which has to be suctioned frequently with a catheter, when he cannot cough up sputum. When too much saliva is in his mouth he needs to be suctioned orally also. He wears a condom catheter, so he does not urinate on himself. He is alert and enjoys watching T.V. He uses voice prosthesis to speak. Every once in a while the feeding becomes dislodged and he has to return to the hospital for placement, and that is when I get to see him. At home, his family takes excellent care of him. He is always clean and has no bed sores. In this case the police did make three arrests. I do not know what happened, but only one of the three went to prison, and he was sentenced to five years. Five years seems a very lenient sentence for ruining some one's life.

THE TOUGH MARINE
She volunteered her live-in boyfriend

When working as a home health care coordinator, (a nurse who reads the doctors discharge orders and coordinates between home health providers, to furnish the care ordered by the doctor) I had to set up home health care for a forty year old woman who fell and lacerated her left thigh playing tackle football with her eighteen year-old nephew on a gravel road. After doing self-treatment at home, the wound became infected. Realizing that the wound was beyond her abilities, the woman went to the emergency room, and was admitted to the hospital. A debridement (removal of infected non-viable material) was performed on the wound and the woman was placed on I.V. antibiotics. Her original discharge plan was to send her home on a wound vac (wound suction device used on wounds where the injury oozes more fluid than a bandage can hold) and I.V. antibiotics. The doctors in charge of her care decided to scrap the original plan, and send her home on oral antibiotics and dressing changes twice a day. The dressing change involved packing the wound with dressing sock soaked in sterile saline, and covering it overall with dry dressings.

When I went up to interview the woman and examine the wound, I noted that she did not have health insurance. I told her the hospital would be willing to provide four free home health care visits by a registered nurse in order to train someone to change the dressings. I asked her if she had any family members who would be capable of performing a dressing change. The woman at first said that she could do her own dressing changes. I told her given the size and location of the wound, I did not think that would work. She next volunteered her live-in boyfriend.

I phoned the man and asked him if he would be willing to change his girlfriend's dressing. I suggested he come to the hospital, and watch a dressing change, before he gives his answer. I explained that the wound was deep and somewhat ugly to look at. He assured me he did not have to go to the hospital for training, that he could perform the dressing changes because he was a US Marine. He gave me the impression that he had a wealth of experience in wounds based on his prior military service. The patient was discharged that evening from the hospital, and the plans were laid to have the home health nurse teach the boyfriend the dressing change routine.

The next day, I received a call from the home health care nurse who was at the patient's house. While she was removing the bandage, with the marine watching, he had an opportunity to see the entire wound exposed. Evidently, the sight overwhelmed his senses and he passed out on the floor. I was very upset, because I told the nurse, I had requested the boyfriend come to the hospital and observe one dressing change, before agreeing to perform his girlfriend's dressing changes. His response was "I don't have to I was a Marine." I told the nurse to kick him in the ass for me, and when he wakes up, he still has to learn to change the dressing. The marine eventually regained consciousness, and after retching a few times, learned how to do a wet to dry dressing change.

WHY HIM, WHY NOT ME TOO

There was no change in his condition

I was working the 3-11 shift at a local hospital. It just so happened that this hospital was selected to do a clinical trial for a clot busting medication to be used on stroke patients. The study was a triple blind study which neither the doctor, the patient or the staff knew if the drug or saline was given to the patient. This means that the patient either got the new medication or nothing to reverse the debilitating symptoms of the stroke. There are pitfalls to this type of study, and this story details one of these cases.

The study mentioned above has been tested many times in many hospitals with miraculous and devastating results for the patients. For the sake of humanity, some studies are terminated, and all patients were given the correct medication because the cure was so dramatic that it was inhumane to continue giving part of the patient population water.

Where I was working, specialists were waiting in the emergency to give the cloaked medications to patients that met certain criterion. For purposes of the study, the stroke had to be witnessed, and the patient had to be brought to the emergency room in less than 45 minutes from onset. For the most part fire rescue was the transport method because of their quick response and their low transport times.

I received two admissions that evening, and both were patients that had come through the emergency room and fit the stroke protocol. Both were administered a cloaked medication by the team in the ER. The first patient I received was 86 years old and in reasonably good physical condition for his advanced age. His mental condition was an issue as he had been suffering from dementia for several years. A family member was with him at the bedside so I was able to complete the admission and resolve any issues immediately apparent. He had complete paralysis on his left side with facial drop and drooling from the corner of his mouth. He was unable to communicate at all and was very drowsy.

About 2 hours later I received another patient from the ER who also fit the stroke protocol. This time it was a 50 year old man who was talking to his wife in the living room when he was stricken. He was awake and alert but was unable to speak due to facial drop on the right side. He had right side paralysis but was very strong on the left side and was able to move around enough to make himself comfortable. His wife was at the bedside but was very upset and barely able to answer the admission questions I had to ask. He was also incontinent of urine and had to be cleaned shortly after being placed in the bed by the ER staff who brought him to the floor.

As the evening progressed, I received visits from the stroke protocol staff to evaluate the two patients at preselected intervals. They would do a specialized assessment on each patient using the study forms. Before the shift was over at 11:00 PM there was a marked improvement in the 86 year old patient. He began to move his arm and fingers, and was able to pull his leg up by bending his knee. I guess you can imagine how the 50 year old was fairing. You guessed it, there was no change in his condition. I left the hospital a little after 11:00PM and returned the following evening.

As usual I was assigned the same patients that I had previously. After taking report from the day nurse, I went to the first patient's room to do my initial assessment. The 86 year old was sitting up in bed watching TV and lightly conversing with relatives in the room. He was able to follow simple commands and had command of his limbs. Everyone was in good spirits, and the family was looking forward to seeing the family physician to question him about a discharge date.

I went to the next patients room, the 50 year old, and

found him in the same condition he had been in the night before. The only addition was a Foley catheter inserted into his bladder through his penis. That was done to preserve his skin integrity from breakdown caused by urine leakage. There were family members in the room, and they were very upset, including two school aged children. I did my assessment, saw nothing urgent to do and proceeded on to my next patient.

Every nurse on the floor realized what had happened with the stroke medications given. The 86 year old got the real medication and the 50 year old received the water. How unfortunate that the only way to get medications approved for widespread administration is to conduct clinical trials like this.

Today, the stroke protocol is in full use, and all patients receive the real medication.

As an aside to this story I should relate a well known issue with clinical trials that happened at a New England mental institution.

A scientist working for a drug company had some success with a drug he was using on large animals in testing. He received permission to do a clinical trial on human patients residing in a mental institution. The medication was being administered in a blind experiment, meaning that no one knew which patient was receiving the medication, and which patient was receiving a sugar pill. Each patient was to be evaluated by a study psychiatrist at pre-selected intervals. Of course, the patients did not know who was getting the medication and who was not. The study progressed for several months without incident until an issue developed when the evaluating psychiatrists got together to review their interim findings. They all found that every one of their patients showed marked improvement in their symptoms. They knew that only some of the patients were given the study medications yet all showed improvement. A decision was made to investigate and report on this phenomenon. It was decided to ask each patient if he or she noticed and difference in their activities and why. There was a consensus that they all felt they were receiving the real medication, and none of them felt they were the one getting the sugar pill. Consequently, all of the patients showed a reduction in their symptoms and were all getting better. The entire patient population was self-curing their mental problems regardless of their diagnosis. The study was a failure and the study medications were discontinued and everything went back the way it was before the study began.

THE MYSTERY MAN

Police did not believe he was prone to escape

As a nurse who spent most of his career working on a telemetry floor, I had a few patients who developed chest pain after being arrested. This is not an unusual ploy. By claiming to have chest pain, the person arrested person postpones going to jail. Instead of taking the person to jail, the police take them to the hospital, where they receive a cardiac workup. A cardiac workup usual takes a day to complete. We draw cardiac enzymes every six hours x three and usually do an echocardiogram. If a person's angina is legitimate, the cardiac enzymes will be elevated. The echocardiogram is an ultra sound of the heart; the purpose is to evaluate heart function. While in the hospital the patient can call his lawyer who can arrange for him to be bonded out once he reaches the county jail. As soon as the doctor says there is nothing wrong with the patient's heart, the police take him to jail where he is met by his lawyer and shortly released.

In my thirty-eight years of nursing almost all arrestees' cardiac workups were negative. In fact, I can remember only one that was positive.

One evening a male who had been arrested was brought to the floor from the E.R. for a cardiac workup. The man was in either his late forties or early fifties. He was nondescript; brown hair, brown eyes and medium built. He was the kind of guy if you put him in a crowd nobody would notice him.

While driving a car the man was stopped by a police officer. The officer thought there was something suspicious about the car and the man driving it. The officer asked to see the man's driver's license and he told the cop that he left it at home. The policeman next ran his license plate number and the plate did not match the car, so an arrest was made. As soon as he was arrested, the man started complaining of chest pain. Instead of going to jail, he went to the E.R. From the E.R. he was transferred to the telemetry floor. His cardiac workup was positive, so he was taken to the cath lab and had a cardiac catheterization with a stent placement (one of his cardiac arteries was blocked). Because he had a cardiac catheterization the police did not believe he was prone to escape, so no guard was put in his room. The day after his stent placement he quietly took off his hospital gown, put on his clothes and went down the backstairs of the telemetry floor. He left the hospital and walked to a nearby used car lot. There he purchased a vehicle with a stolen check. He must have been a first rate con-artist because he got a used car dealer to accept a phony check.

After purchasing the car he drove off. Nobody knows the man's real name (he gave a false name when admitted) or where he went. He had no visitors when he was in the hospital and made no telephone calls (this was before cell phones, so calls would have to be made from his hospital room phone). As far as I know he was never rearrested by the police, nor was the newly purchased used car ever recovered. He remains a mystery.

SHIT IN A CAN

Nutritional condition was bordering on starvation

Doctors admit patients to the hospital for thousands of ailments, some ailments are mysteries that are never solved, and some are so simple that they are missed completely by everyone. In this case, a routine office visit and blood test produced a result that caught everyone by surprise. When the doctor reviewed an elderly male's blood test the day after his visit, he called the man at home and had him report to the hospital for a direct admission. (an admission that goes directly to the floor, not through the emergency room) I was assigned the gentleman who was puzzled as to why the doctor was sending him in to be admitted. The doctor noted that he would be in to write the orders on the man when the office closed for the day. (this was not unusual).

When the doctor arrived, he ordered a battery of tests and scans to be conducted over the next two days, so the gentleman was out of the room for most of my next two shifts, returning only to eat and to sleep. This centered around a very poor result in one of the blood tests, telling the doctor that the gentleman's nutritional condition was bordering on starvation. He was of smaller thin stature, but was able to walk, talk, and was lucid, so I could see that when he was dressed, he would look fine. The doctor began looking for something that would rob him of his nutrition.

All of the tests came back OK no culprit revealed itself, and a subsequent blood test revealed a marked change in his test results for the better, so the patient was discharged on the forth day after supper when the doctor came by, with a three-month follow-up in the office. The patient kept the appointment, and his blood test again revealed ultra-poor nutritional status, returning to where he was during the initial hospitalization.

Again, the patient was admitted, the doctor felt that he had missed something on the first round of tests. During the admission, the patient revealed that six month's ago his wife had died, and he missed her very much. He also remarked what a great cook she was, and how he missed her wonderful meals. I asked him who was now preparing his food for him, or was he doing it himself. He reported that he had never prepared a meal, that he had seen on TV that he could get all the proper nutrition in a can. He had gone to the supermarket and purchased several cases of a nutritional drink called BOOST. He was drinking one for breakfast, one for lunch, and two for supper.

Everything became clear immediately why he was starving to death. He got regular food on his last admission, so his nutritional status got better. He returned home on the BOOST diet, and his nutritional status returned to very poor again. The problem was solved, so I left a note for the doctor on the patient's chart.

The doctor ordered home health with an aide and dietitian to call on the gentleman. They would take him to the store, and show him how to make and prepare better choices, and get him enrolled in Meals on Wheels where he would get meals sent to his home.

SHE THOUGHT SHE KNEW EVERYTHING
I couldn't believe the physician would go ahead

Arrogance in medicine will only get you in trouble. Also, there is a difference between knowing, and assuming. I was the administrator of an out-patient surgical center that employed seven RN's. I worked alongside them daily, and had confidence in their abilities. Our tasks were to admit the patients, assess their physical condition, place them on a heart monitor, and place an IV for sedation. An operative permit was also signed by the patient to give permission for the procedure. Once this was accomplished, the doctor was called, the nurse anesthetist would interview the patient, and the patient was taken to the procedure room where an RN would monitor the patient during the procedure.

On this day a patient kept her appointment even though she was sick with an upper respiratory infection. The RN admitting the patient identified the problem right away by listening to her lungs as her part of the initial assessment. Once she spotted the complication, she stopped the admitting process. The RN rightfully halted the procedure and notified me to take a look at her patient to confirm her findings. I introduced my self to the patient and asked her how long she had been sick, she replied three or four days. After listening to her lungs, I agreed with the initial findings and decided that we would not continue with the admission. The patient had a sedation order, and I felt that it was too dangerous to sedate that patient. We left the patient in the prep area and called the physician with our findings.

After a few minutes the physician came to see the patient. He talked with the patient, and asked the nurse anesthetist to examine the patient. She talked with the patient, while I talked with the physician. I explained the issue to the physician, and he said he would go with whatever the nurse anesthetist decided. I then told him that I would not allow our staff to assist in the case regardless of what the nurse anesthetist decided. I said my responsibility is to protect the surgical center from liability, and to protect the patient from harm, therefore we would have no part in any procedure on that patient. (since the doctor had a piece of the surgical center, I could not stop him from using the building and contents, but all of the liability would be his) What we had was a Mexican Standoff, seven nurses and the administrator against the nurse anesthetist and the doctor. The nurse anesthetist had deemed the patient acceptable, and had placed the IV and attached the patient to the monitor. Since she never admitted patients, she forgot to get the permit signed or to complete the necessary paperwork that had been started by my staff. My staff was instructed that anything she did with the patient was her responsibility, we were totally hands-off at that point. The admission, the procedure and the recovery and discharge of the patient was the sole responsibility of the doctor and the nurse anesthetist. This was unusual, and had never happened before, and I couldn't believe that the physician would go ahead with a procedure under those conditions, but he did.

The patient was taken to the procedure room and prepared by the nurse anesthetist and she began to administer the anesthesia. The patient went asleep, and in three minutes went into respiratory arrest. The nurse anesthetist hit the code button, and her supervising physician was called from an adjacent building. All hell broke loose, as I immediately called 911 on the telephone and requested a fire rescue squad. The anesthesiologist placed a breathing tube in the patient's airway and began oxygenating the patient, saving the day. The patient was stable on the monitor, and her vital signs were elevated but OK.

When I told the anesthesiologist that the rescue was in route, he said that he wanted to "pull the breathing tube" before they arrived. I refused to let him do that, telling him that, "you had better be able to replace it in a hurry if she arrests when the tube is pulled, I don't recommend it." Rescue arrived, and the patient was removed to the hospital where she remained for over a week in intensive care. Both doctors involved visited her every day while she was hospitalized. Additionally, they were informed that the patient had never signed the permission slips for either the procedure or the anesthesia, so they were doubly liable for everything. Lucky for them a lawyer was never involved in the case. The cocky nurse anesthetist, was in the opinion of the nursing staff mentally ill, and went on to get herself in other jambs as my tenure there wore on. We watched her like a hawk, and went "hands off" several other times during our tenure there. I also talked to her supervising physician about our concerns and documented our talk in notes kept in the office. If anything serious ever transpired, and a lawyer was involved, I was prepared to throw both of them "under the bus."

TAKE YOUR CHANCES 3 STORIES
The doctor lost his lawsuit

My entire nursing career has been spent working in Florida. Although most of the doctors I worked with I liked, and respected, Florida has more than its share of bad physicians. I believe the reason for this is because it is a transient state. Most people are not born here, but come from other states. When people arrive here, they do not know anyone. In their home state if they needed a physician they would ask friends or relatives for recommendations, so they would know who to avoid. If a doctor cannot make it in his home state because of a lack of competency, come to Florida where knows body knows you. This works not only for medicine, but other occupations. Another reason marginally competent physicians can flourish in Florida, is most of their patients are elderly. The elderly, tend to view all people who have M.D. or DO after their name as Gods.

One day I was working the evening shift (3-11 PM) in I.C.U. I normally worked on the telemetry floor, but that day I floated to I.C.U. One of the two patients I was taking care of was a post-op who had a new colostomy. Colostomy is the opening of some portion of the colon through the abdominal wall. Colostomies divert the flow of stool from its normal route, out of the colon into a bag attached to the skin at the colostomy site. The bag is usually emptied once a day. The bag is changed every three to seven days. There are several reasons for a colostomy: colon cancer, trauma to the bowel, Crohn's Disease, Diverticulitis, bowel obstruction, and bowel incontinence.

There are some surgeons that you never have a problem with their patients. They have no post-op complications. On the other hand, some surgeons if you get assigned their patients you can guarantee there are going to be complications. This patient had one of those surgeons whose patients almost always had complications. When I received the patient at 3PM he was alert and orientated, and his vital signs were stable. Within four hours he was confused and hypotensive (low blood pressure) with a rapid heartbeat. The first sign of hemorrhage is mental confusion (not enough blood carrying oxygen going to the brain). Due to the loss of blood, the blood pressure drops and the body tries to compensate for the loss of blood by beating faster.

I emptied the colostomy bag which was filled with blood, so I called the doctor. I informed him of the situation and told him I emptied a colostomy bag filled with blood. His response was "are you sure it is blood"? I replied "well it was red, viscous and smelled like blood. I did not taste it, so I do not know if it tasted like blood." He told me he would be right over to see the patient. To ensure blood got to his brain, I put the patient in Trendelenburg (a head down feet up position). Next to elevate his blood pressure I ran I.V. fluid as fast as possible into him.

To his credit, within minutes of calling him, the doctor was on the unit and within an hour the patient had returned to the operating room. My shift ended while the patient was still in surgery, so I do not know the outcome of the operation or why the patient hemorrhaged, but I'm sure the doctor found out..

At the same hospital I took care of the patient of another physician who had less than a stellar reputation. The patient in question was an attractive young lady who had a colon resection with anastomosis. A colon resection with anastomosis is where part of the colon is surgically removed and the two remaining ends are then reconnected, allowing fecal matter to pass through the colon and out the rectum. The reconnection is done with either sutures or staples. The operation is done to remove a diseased part of the colon or a blockage. Think of it as if you had a water pipe and there was a blockage. You cut into the pipe where the blockage is and remove that part of the pipe that is blocked and then reattach the open ends so water can flow through the pipe.

I had this surgery myself and spent three days in the hospital before being discharged home, so I knew there was something wrong when this patient was in the hospital for six days. She had a nasogastric tube (going from the nose into the stomach) suctioning out gastric contents. Every time the tube was pulled the patient became nauseated. When I had my surgery, I was nauseated the first day post-op. By the second day I was eating green Jello, on the third day I was passing liquid stool and was discharged.

After almost two weeks in the hospital, the young lady's surgeon consulted another surgeon (the same doctor who did my surgery). It was discovered that he did not reconnect the two opened ends of the colon. Instead he sewed an open end of the colon to the side of the same colon, so stomach contents could not move out of the stomach. The woman went through a second operation. This time the colon was correctly reconnected. The lady made a speedy recovery and four days later was discharged. Shortly after this fiasco, her surgeon (first operation) announced he was giving up the practice of medicine and going to law school. The nurses started joking "soon he will be able to defend his own malpractice suits."

A PARIAH

Doctors rarely bring complaints about another physician

I worked at a hospital where there was a cardiac surgeon who was so bad that the operating room nurses refused to work with him. The scrub nurse is the nurse in the operating room who hands the surgeon instruments, helps with applying dressings to the incision and makes sure the operating room is clean before the surgical procedure begins. Before the operation begins the scrub nurse counts all the instruments, needles and sponges. After the operation before the surgeon closes the scrub nurse recounts the instruments, needles and sponges to make sure nothing has been left inside the patient.

Besides the scrub nurse there is also a circulating nurse in operating room. The circulating nurse does a second count of the equipment (she double checks the scrub nurse's count before and after the operation). She also does the charting in surgery, gets addition supplies if needed and serves as a patient advocate.

In response to the refusal of the operating room nurses to work with him, the doctor hired his own nurses to work in the OR. Finally, he lost his privileges, after two of his fellow cardiac surgeons complained about him to hospital administration. Doctors rarely bring complaints about another physician. In my thirty-eight years in nursing I have known only six physicians who lost hospital privileges. The surgeon who lost privileges sued the two doctors who complained about him, for restraint of trade. During the trial it came out, the surgeon in question had a 19% mortality rate. That meant 19% of his open heart patients died on the operating table. The national average was a 5.5% mortality rate for open heart operations. It was also revealed that the man was not a board certified cardiac surgeon, so I cannot figure out why the hospital was allowing him to perform open heart surgery.

Needless to say, the doctor lost his lawsuit. He ended up closing his practice and moving to Texas. I am not sure if he continued to practice medicine. During the trial, one of the doctors I liked and respected told me he knows two physicians he would like to see lose their privileges, but he has not lodged complaints because he does not want to get sued.

After the trial, one of the nurses I worked with told me that her mother was a patient of the above surgeon and died on the operating table undergoing open heart surgery. She also told me that she wonders had another surgeon operated on her mother would she be alive today. I asked her why her mother picked this surgeon. She told me her parents just moved down from Michigan and did not know any doctors in Florida.

RICH PEOPLE'S LIVES

All they did was order out from a stack of menu's

Even rich people get sick. I was sent to an exclusive development on the outskirts of one of the larger cities in Florida. This development was surrounding an exclusive golf course. The homes were all custom multi story affairs looking like each owner was trying to outdo the neighbor in opulence. There is a wall around the complete perimeter allowing entrance and exit only through a gated guard post manned by a private security guard. I announced who I was visiting, a call was made, and I was admitted and given directions to which tree lined lane I was to use to get to the mansion. These homes were the property of very wealthy people, including four-star generals, professional sports coaches, and owners of very large distributorships. The house was visible from the street, and was not a traditional house that you would think a very wealthy person would live in. It was a two story affair, something that an architect would live in, sort of an architect gone wild, approach to housing, with large two story arches across the front.

I was directed to park out of the way of the four garage doors, on the side where a delivery van was parked. (the van was used by a servant to go to the store for the couple who lived there). One garage door was raised for me, and I entered the house through the garage which after passing through another door found me in a dining room adjacent to the kitchen. The lady of the house met me there and directed me to set up my iv's in that dining room. I was asked if I had brought my lunch, and I said I had (I would be there all day). She said that I had two options, I could use the refrigerator in the pool kitchen, or the one in the garage next to the door I had entered through. She also said that the refrigerator in the garage was full of soft drinks and I could have anything I desired. (I didn't drink soft drinks, I brought my own iced tea) The couple were sitting at a little café type table at a large window overlooking the pool. They were having morning coffee and eating some Danish. I set about preparing my iv infusion for the gentleman. He had a port which was already accessed, so I just plugged in the IV and hung the bag from a rolling IV pole next to his chair. I had to walk through the kitchen to get to him.

The kitchen was a medium sized kitchen exceptionally well equipped. I remember two stainless side-by-side refrigerators, and a large eight burner restaurant quality stove with a grill to one side. You could prepare almost anything in that kitchen. After I hooked up the IV I took my lunch and put it into the refrigerator in the pool cabana, which also had a full stainless kitchen with ice maker. I had to get something from the car, so I went back through the garage where a custom golf cart and classic Lincoln coupe sat in two of the four bays. When I returned, the wife said "I'll be upstairs in the gym if you need me for something", and left. The husband told me he was going to lie down and pointed toward a doorway on the right side of a two-story fireplace across a quite large recreation room filled with leather chairs and sofas.

While I was making up additional IV in the small dining room (there was a larger dining room which sat about twelve people within sight of the smaller one) a grocery man came in through the same door to the garage I entered. He had a hand truck with boxes of food stacked on it. He went directly over to one of the stainless refrigerators and started emptying it of everything. He then took everything in the boxes and replaced everything he had removed with new food. I was astonished, I saw lobster, shrimp, steaks, every type of vegetable, liquids like cream, milk, and juices go. The same things were replenished, and the grocer left taking everything back out on the hand truck. When the wife came down from her exercise room, I told her what had transpired. I said that all the food he removed looked good to me, should he really have removed it all? She replied "well, he has to make a living too, doesn't he?" I thought it was wasteful because while I was there for the day, all they did was order out from a stack of menu's the wife had on her side of the table.

I went into the bedroom to take down the old bag and begin infusing the next IV bag. The husband was sitting up in an enormous bed reading with his glasses on. I took down the IV and plugged in the new one and left the room. I was shocked by what was in the room. He had a large desk, with two large couches facing each other in front of the desk. There was a small set of book shelves behind the desk on the wall full of books and papers. There were floor lamps at each end of the couches with a large oriental rug on the floor under the desk and couches, and all of this in an enormous bedroom. Alongside the bed on the left was a door which led to a large bathroom and dressing room closet, and another doorway which led to his wife's bathroom and dressing room closet and her bedroom. All of this behind the enormous fireplace which went up two stories and through the roof.

This was not the only wealthy home I had been in and they all had the same thing in common. The couples spent their time sitting by a window in a small cozy spot in their homes. These gigantic homes were almost totally unused except for a little well worn area next to a window where they preferred to sit together. I remember approaching another mansion with very unkept lawn and shrubs, the house needing paint, and care. When I went inside it was a mess, the pool table had newspapers and trash all over it. The large TV on the wall was dark, and the people were watching a little 12 in. portable in their little sitting area surrounded with clutter. I made my visit, and left wondering how such wealthy people had mismanaged their lives to get in that state.

I went to a home right on the beach where a widower multimillionaire lived, and both he and his female caretaker were eating something out of cans that looked like dogfood. The caretaker did not know how to cook, and refused to let another woman into the house. Only men could provide care to the patient which had a debilitating stroke and was paralyzed. The caretaker was terrified that if the patient was near another woman, he would take a liking to her, so she kept him isolated from any other women. Her fear was based on the fact that that was how she came to live with the multimillionaire. Additionally, he was non-verbal and had dementia. They never went out anywhere, and a relative shopped for them from a list the caretaker provided. They bought rotisserie chickens from the supermarket, and canned Vienna sausages which the caretaker peeled every morning for them to eat. They lived a strange life where money did them no good what so ever, his Mercedes and her Cadillac were rotting dust covered in the garage. I lived much better than they did on a fraction of the income.

ON THE CHEAP

He hooked up to the hospitals water system

While working as a home health care coordinator I had a male patient who had a total knee replacement. The man had really bad insurance (the kind that does not pay much for home care). I had a difficult time finding an agency that would accept this man. His care required a nurse to change his dressing three times a week and physical therapy three times a week. After three days, I finally found an agency that agreed to accept the case. I walked triumphantly into the patient's room. The man was very happy, he told me that he was being discharged later that day. I told him no problem, I found a home care agency and they could start tomorrow. His response was, "but you do not know where to send them." I responded, "are you not going to be at your house in Saint Petersburg." He said "no I am going to be in your parking lot." He proceeded to tell me the day before his surgery he and his wife drove their large motor home to the hospital and parked in the main employee parking lot. Being a home health care coordinator I parked in the administrative parking lot, so I hadn't seen it.. He told me his wife has been living in the parking lot since his surgery, and they planned another two weeks in the parking lot before going home. He told me that his large motor home was parked by the security guard's shack and he was able to hookup to the electricity from the shack and he also hooked up to the hospital's water system.

I told him that he could not stay in the main employee parking lot. First of all, there is barely enough parking spaces for employees. Next there is the liability. He assured me his wife was safe and that every two hours a security guard's car came by the motor home on patrol. I thought to myself

"I guess hospital security must think it is normal to have a motor home parked in the employee parking lot." This shows the quality of hospital security. Nobody investigated a strange vehicle using hospital electricity.

I called my boss and informed her of the situation. She called the D.O.N. (director of nursing). The D.O.N. came up to the patient's room and told him he could not live in the parking lot. The patient's daughter ended up driving him, his wife and their motor home back to Saint Petersburg, where he received his home health care.

Later I found out not only did the man own a $100,000 motor home, and a house in St. Petersburg, but he also he had a condo out on the beach. Even a small one bedroom condo on the beach, would cost considerable money. This gives one an idea of the man's priorities, it was not his health, or health insurance. He spent money on all this unnecessary stuff and got the cheapest health insurance he could buy.

LISTEN UP!

For the third time I went over the discharge instructions

In speaking to patients, they often hear only what they want to hear. This causes many problems. When a patient is admitted to the hospital, the admitting physician will often consult other physicians. For example, if a patient comes in with chest pain, the admitting physician will consult a cardiologist. Today a patient may have two or three consults. That patient with chest pain might also be in kidney failure, so nephrologists may also be consulted. The admitting physician is the primary physician, and is in charge of the patient's over all care. The admitting physician, or if he has the day off, the physician covering for him, can only discharge the patient. Something common is that a consulting physician will come in and tell a patient that from his point of view he can be discharged. Often the patient will start getting dressed. He will call for the nurse and say that he has been discharged. The nurse then would explain to the patient that the primary physician has to discharge him; the consulting doctor cannot discharge you. The patient will repeat that the doctor (consultant) has told him he can be discharged, the nurse will have to repeat the explanation. Many times, the explanation must be done three times before the patient understands what he was being told to him.

Sometimes a primary physician will write conditional discharge orders. The conditional discharge orders will say that a patient may be discharge if the consulting physicians agree to the discharge. Again, the patient does not hear that his discharge depends on the consulting physicians agreeing to his release, so the nurse must go in and explain to the patient the conditions of his discharge, at least twice.

Because patients hear only what they want to hear, when

I give discharge instructions, I like the spouse to be there. So, what one person misses the other person may pick up. I started doing this when I had a patient return to the hospital two days after being discharged. The woman was discharged with a prescription for nitroglycerin. I explained to her the drug was to be taken for chest pain. The patient only heard pain. Two days later she was having back pain, so she took the nitroglycerin. The pill did not relieve her back pain, so she took another pill. She remembered that she could take up to three nitroglycerin pills for pain. The second tablet did not relieve the pain, so she took a third. Nitroglycerin is a vasodilator. A vasodilator increases the size of the blood vessels. This causes the blood pressure to drop. This drop in blood pressure caused the patient to pass out. The woman landed on her face which caused her to have two black eyes.

Sometimes having two persons listening to discharge instruction does not work either. I had a patient who the discharging physician spent fifteen minutes with a patient and his wife explaining his discharge instructions. After the doctor was finish, I explained the discharge instructions for a second time. Later that day I received a telephone call from the patient's wife. She had questions about the discharge instruction, so I went over the instructions for the second time. The next morning, I received a second call from the wife regarding her husband's discharge instructions. For the third time, I went over the discharge instruction. This wife had the discharge instructions explained to her a total of four times before she heard the entirety of the instructions.

This selective hearing is not limited to discharge. I worked with a nurse who had an elderly post op. patient. The patient had orders to be up in a chair. The nurse came into the room and told the patient he was there to get her up into the chair. The patient refused. The nurse then asked the patient "what nursing home do you plan to go to when you are discharged." The woman said that "I am not going to a nursing home, I am going home." The nurse responded "not unless you get out of bed and start moving." Well the woman did not hear "unless you get out of bed and start moving." When the woman's son came to visit, she told him that "the nurse said I am going to a nursing home when I am discharged." The son became enraged, stormed out of the patient's room and demanded to speak to the nurse manager. If the patient did not have selective hearing, this problem would have been avoided.

IT'S THE NURSES FAULT
He tried to force the NG tube

As a nurse, one thing you learn is that if there is a screw up in the hospital it is assumed that it is the nurse's fault. Even if a nurse had nothing to do with the event, it is assumed a nurse screwed up. This is reinforced by T.V. and the movies. In T.V. and the movies, doctors are gods, nurses are mere humans. Gods do not make mistakes.

One Sunday afternoon, while working in N.I.C.U.(neuro-intensive care unit) we received a new admit from the E.R. She was a woman in her late fifties who suffered a stroke. Nothing unusual in this, but what was unusual was her family doctor came up to the unit with her when she was being transferred from the E.R. to intensive care. Normally in a case like this, if the family doctor is called, he will see the patient in the E.R. In the E.R., he will examine the patient, write orders and then leave. The next day they will see the patient in the unit.

Once we got the patient settled on the floor (moved the patient from stretcher to a bed, took vital signs and performed a brief physical assessment) the family doctor told us he was going to insert an N.G. tube (nasogastric tube). This is a plastic tube that is inserted through the nostril, down the esophagus and into the stomach. This tube is used to suction gastric contents out of the stomach or it can be used to feed patients. Inserting a N.G. tube is one of those procedures like; inserting a urinary catheter, an I.V. or pulling a central line that is usually done by an R.N.

I do not like inserting N.G. tubes. The process is very uncomfortable for the patient and they usually try to fight you. There is also a good chance that the tube will be inserted in the lung. If the patient starts coughing a lot after insertion, the tube is probably in the lung and has to be removed and reinserted. One way you know if the tube is in the stomach is gastric content comes out of the tube. Another way is with an air bolus. You take a 60 ML syringe filled with air insert it into the top of the tube and push the plunger down while listening to bowel sounds with a stethoscope. If you hear a swish sound in the stomach, you are fairly certain the tube is in the right place. The tube is then secured by taping it to the nose. Before using the tube to feed the patient an x-ray is taken to confirm placement. I know of a case where a nurse gave the patient liquid potassium down a N.G. tube before getting an x-ray and the tube was in the lung. This resulted in lung damage for the patient.

Sometimes the N.G. tube cannot be advanced past the nostril. I never try to force the tube. Once I meet resistance I stop, and try the other nostril. If unable to insert through either nostril, I inform the doctor the tube was unable to be inserted. The doctor will then usually order the patient to be taken to x-ray and the radiologist will try to insert the tube.

This family doctor began inserting the N.G. tube. I am not sure why he felt the patient needed an N.G. tube. Her stomach was not distended. Normally we would start the patient on I.V. fluids and consult speech therapy for a swallowing evaluation before inserting an N.G. tube.

While inserting the tube the doctor met resistance, instead of stopping he tried to force the N. G. tube through the nose. He stopped when the patient started bleeding, then it was up to the nurses to stop the bleeding. He turned around walked over to the nurse's station and sat down. When we told him we were having difficulty in stopping the bleeding, he told us to page the E.N.T. (ear nose and throat doctor) on call. We did and the E.N.T. promptly came to the unit and examined the patient. In a loud voice the E.N.T. stated "I would like to meet the dumb-ass nurse who tried to insert this N.G. tube. The patient has a deviated septum." He also said, " I would like to know why it was so important to insert this N.G. tube?" The nurses turned around and stared at the family doctor. He looked like a deer caught in headlights. He quietly slinked out of the N.I.C.U., but before he left, he consulted a neurologist. As far as I know he never returned to the N.I.C.U. while the woman was in the unit.

The woman spent three days in the N.I.C.U., and then she was transferred to the neurology floor. After two weeks on the neurology floor she was transferred to rehab. It is interesting that the E.N.T. assumed that a nurse tried to insert the N.G. tube and that the family doctor never corrected him.

THE DO OVER

He went into a coma that night

While working the telemetry floor at a local hospital I encountered an older gentleman who was bedridden, and dying of terminal cancer. He was one of the nicer patients I had, and I enjoyed conversing with him when I had a short interval between my tasks. Always present in his room during visiting hours was a woman about his age that I just assumed was his wife. I found out several days later that the frequent visitor was a neighbor. He was admitted to the hospital because he lived alone, and there was no one to provide the full time care he required as his life was coming to an end.

Several days from his death, there was a flurry of visitors that came to see him, namely a younger man and woman, who during his illness I had not seen before. The only daily visitor was the older woman. With all the activity in the room, the older lady left almost as if the younger couple pushed her out. They hovered and smothered him with. "let me fix that for you" or "let me adjust this for you" while they visited that day, and then they were gone. The next day the older lady returned, and things settled down just as they were before.

Early that night, I had a chance to visit his room, and he signaled that he wanted to talk. He told me that he had no children with his wife, who had died years before. He reported that the younger visitors were his brother's children who he had not seen in the last 15 years. He said that while they were in the room, all they talked about was money. They asked him what he thought his home was worth, where he banked, what kind of car he had, etc. He knew that they had a copy of his will which left everything to his brother. Since the brother had recently died, they were to become the beneficiaries of his will, and that was why they rushed to see him. They made notes while they were there so they could access their windfall with a minimum of time spent in Florida, since they didn't live there.

The old man began to reflect on his past twenty years without his wife, and how he developed a relationship with his neighbor which began with him offering to drive her to an appointment. The neighbor reciprocated by cooking him dinner that night, and helping him with his wash. The relationship persisted for twenty years, however, each of them stayed in their own homes, but they cooperated and helped each other every day. He remarked that he was so sad to be dying and the old lady he loved so much would get nothing to remember him by. He said to me "I wish I could do things over, I wish I had left everything to my dearest friend." I asked him if he had a lawyer and he said yes and spouted his name out right away. I said "I'll be right back", and left the room. I went directly to the phone in the nurses station, and called information, and got the lawyer's phone number, and called him. I was able after several minutes, to talk directly to the lawyer, and explained that I was a nurse in the hospital, and told him all the particulars surrounding the dying man. The lawyer said that he would bring a blank will to the hospital that very night and visit with the old man.

After supper trays were collected, down the hall came a man in a suit with a briefcase, and went into the old man's room. After about an hour he exited the room, came over to me and thanked me for calling him, he said that this was one of the cases that made him happy he had become a lawyer. Later I visited the old man and he was ecstatic, he said that now he could die in peace, he was so happy that his friend would have an easier life because of him. He thanked me for helping him, and settled down for a long sleep. He went into a coma that night and never awakened again. He was in the coma for 24 hours when a doctor came up to me and told me he was taking the old man downstairs to do a colonoscopy on him. I angrily stated that the patient was on his deathbed and there was nothing to be gained at this late date by doing a colonoscopy on him. The doctor persisted, and even assisted the aide in getting the comatose man onto a stretcher he had brought with him. After the patient was loaded, they both pushed the patient onto the elevator and disappeared. A few moments later, the elevator doors opened, and who was on the elevator but the doctor, the aide, and a dead old man on the stretcher, he had died in the elevator on the way down. The doctor was pissed and was heard to remark "I really wanted that colonoscopy before he died God dam it."

THE SWEETEST GIRL

Despite all of this, she was always pleasant

When working as a nurse I have come across many memorable patients, one of which was a mildly retarded girl. She was twenty-seven years old and lived in a group home until she had abdominal surgery for a serious case of Crohn's disease. These surgeries are very challenging because there is a fine line between removing not enough small intestine, or too much small intestine. The disease causes weak spots in the wall of the intestine which makes an outpouching called a fistula. Fistulas drain large amounts of small intestine contents from a surgical opening made in the abdomen called an Ileostomy. The fistula was constantly draining and a sizeable bag put over the opening. The surgery was done at a hospital in a neighboring county. Because of her constantly draining fistula she could not go back to her group home and was placed in a nursing home close to the hospital where I worked. The attached bag seemed to always leak and once a month Julie used to come into the hospital with excoriated skin or an infection. The drainage was so copious that we had the ileostomy bag hooked up to wall suction. Despite all this, she was always pleasant. She would call us when her ileostomy bag started to leak and let us know she was wet. She would come to the hospital with her stuffed animals. Each animal had a name and we put hospital bands on her animals.

Once when taking care of her, I mentioned I had a pet cat. She told me that when she was younger, she had a cat that was hit by a car and died. I told her my cat Precious was not doing well, she was suffering from hyperthyroidism and was refusing to take her medicine. This upset the young lady. The next time she was admitted to the hospital, I had the day off.

She asked the nurse who was caring for her, how Precious the Cat was doing. She told the nurse that she was worried about Precious and was praying for her. Her nurse called me at home and informed me of the young lady's worries. I told the nurse to tell her Precious was doing much better and she was taking her medicine. This girl who was so sick was concerned about my cat. The next day when I returned to work, I thanked her for her prayers. She was shortly released and returned to her nursing home. Approximately a month later she was readmitted with a diagnosis of sepsis. While trying to insert a central line, she coded and died, she was still 27 years old.

I often wonder why this sweet soul, who never hurt anyone had to suffer so much. It does not seem fair that this girl had to suffer, while many of the bastards in this world appear to live charmed lives.

HALF EMPTY x2
No sign of cognitive function

I received a patient from surgical ICU at the beginning of my shift. When this happens, the nurse in ICU gives report to the receiving RN before the patient is moved to the new location. From what she told me this was a very sad case.

The patient and his wife both owned independent businesses. She had a beauty salon operated from her home, and he was a website developer who also worked from home. They were watching TV at night when the husband developed a terrible headache. He tried various over the counter medications, but could not get relief, so they headed to the local emergency room. They were seen at the ER and the husband was medicated, which made him feel somewhat better, but the headache was not totally resolved. He received a prescription, and went to a 24 hour pharmacy to get it filled. After getting and taking the medication, they returned home, but the headache persisted. After several hours, the husband returned to the ER because the headache was worse than before, so bad that he could not open his eyes, and had trouble communicating. The ER doctor suspected a problem that a neurologist should handle, so, one was summoned from home to see the patient.

When the neurologist responded he immediately ordered a CT of the head, and called in the on call operating room staff. The patient went comatose while in the CT scanner, so some life support measures were put on standby while the OR was readied. The patient received a craniotomy, (his skull was opened) and it was discovered that he had ruptured an artery in his brain. The neurosurgeon removed half of his brain to get to the ruptured vessel and sealed it off. The patients head was closed, and he was moved into surgical ICU for one to one care (one nurse one patient).

The patient remained in the ICU for a week when a decision was made to move him to a telemetry unit, and I received report on him, revealing the above information. About a half hour after repor,t I received the patient accompanied by his wife, who had been at the bedside throughout. The patient and his wife were both in their middle forties, and in good physical condition. The patient was placed into a private room, and I began my examination. I noticed that he had a lot of hospital-based skin issues, namely bed sores. He had one on the back of his head, both heels, and the base of his spine. After receiving a week of one to one care, this was inexcusable. I set to work floating his heels, (keeping them off the bed) and turned him to his side bolstering him with pillows. (He became a turn and baste patient right away) He was in a coma, and there was no sign of cognitive function at all. As in all comatose patients, he sighed, made some audible verbal noises, and gave the layman the impression that these were positive signs.

Upon hearing these noises, the patients wife became very excited and started calling friends telling them that he was coming to. This put me in a bad spot, do I tell her the truth, that he is functioning on brain stem only, which controls heart beat and breathing, or let her go on believing he is waking up. I made a decision to keep my mouth shut, because I had a strong feeling that she would reject anything I told her anyway. I thought that the doctor would have to do the dirty work if in fact he had not done so already.

The patient remained on my unit for a week, and plans were set in motion to place him in a warehouse type medical arrangement where comatose patients live out the rest of their lives. When the subject was broached to the wife, she refused all talk of sending him there, because she wanted to take him home and care for him herself. I spent several days more training her on the care necessary for his survival outside the hospital, and he was discharged home with his wife providing the care.

There are cases released from hospitals where the wife supplies all the care, and a nurse comes into the home several times a week to train the family of new procedures, or to follow-up on the care the family provides.

A SHELL

This is not her husband

In this case I was assigned to visit a condo where the wife was providing care for another comatose patient. The husband had experienced a severe stroke and was functioning on his brain stem only, there was no sign of any cognitive function. In this case there was a Foley catheter in his bladder, and an IV line through a port in his chest. He was in a special bed to preserve his skin without the continual turning necessary. His wife was providing good care, but was depressed because this was not the man she knew. The man she knew was struck down at home and this person was what she got back from the hospital after they pushed him out. She asked me "how long can he live like this." I told her that he could live a long time if the care we were providing was successful. She reiterated that this was not her husband, and what could she do to hasten his death. I had heard this before from loved ones, so I was not shocked in any way. I gave her general medical information that anyone could get on line, or from many sources. I told her that a human in good physical condition could last about 7 days without water, and a sick person about 5 days. I was referring to the IV bags that were hanging on the IV pole next to his special bed.

After I left the house, she turned off the IV fluids. I came back two days later, and the urine was still flowing but was dark in color and the IV fluids were off. I reviewed his condition, his skin was intact, and everything was within normal parameters. I came back two days later, and removed the Foley catheter because there was no urine flowing for over a day. On the evening of the fifth day I received a call that there was no need to return to the condo, the patient had died.

HIV 2 STORIES

They were both engaging in risky behavior

A.I.D.S. is not the disease that monopolizes the news today, but back in the 90's it was a minor epidemic that made all the news broadcasts. To those of you that are too young to remember, an airline steward contracted the disease in Haiti and spread it throughout the US by visiting gay bathhouses all over the country. Indiscriminate male sexual contacts were the rage in the gay community at the time, but it was soon put out of fashion by the spread of the disease among gay men.

I was working on a wing in a local hospital when the first gay male patient was admitted to spend his final days. Of course, I was assigned the patient, and it began my first exposure to the ravages of the disease. I knew that it was highly contagious if you came in contact with the patient's body fluids. Of course, there is something called Universal Precautions which nurses use which is supposed to protect the nurse from contracting the diseases the patients bring to the hospital. During the A.I.D.S. surge, Universal Precaution seemed to me like crap, I felt fully exposed to the disease, and vulnerable.

The patient was a young male in his 20's, and was brought in virtually comatose, and on his last legs. He was oozing various liquids from lesions all over his body, he had constant discharge from his rectum, and a catheter protruding from his bladder. He was also needing some suction, because of a pneumonia, he was a mess. He required almost one to one care which meant I had to spend a lot of time in his room dodging coughed up sputum, and I was very wary because I had just read a story about a hospice nurse contracting A.I.D.S. from a patient. I think at the time, I would rather face down a gang member than render care to this guy. I kept thinking that I was risking everything for $12.00 an hour salary. (I was right out of school) I completed my shift and went home, threw my uniform and shoes in the trash, and took a long hot shower. When I didn't contract anything six months later, I was elated.

The next A.I.D.S. case was when I was doing home health. I was sent to an apartment to administer IV antibiotics to another young man in his late 20's who again suffered all the issues prevalent with the first patient. The only difference was that he was still walking around and talking. He was living with his mother, who came to town to take care of her son. The son's male lover was visiting him, and they were intertwined on the couch watching TV. I set up on the dining room table, and when I was ready, had the patient come over near the table so I could plug him into the IV bag. I had to wait an hour for the infusion to complete, so I just sat nearby and waited so I could disconnect. I was struck that his lover must have thought that he was immune to the disease, or he possibly had it too. They were both engaging in risky behavior while the visit continued, like kissing, and massaging each other. (there were open lesions present)

I asked the mother if she had been schooled on what precautions to take, and she reported that she had. I asked her what duties she performed for her son, and she stated that she shopped, cooked, and cleaned and washed clothes, all domestic stuff. I wrapped the visit up as soon as I could, and got out of there, with the two guys back to their hugging and kissing again. I was stunned because the patient had open lesions all over his face, what could they be thinking of? In any case, things got much better for A.I.D.S. cases after gay doctors, and researchers became infected. They soon developed protocols to treat the disease because I know both a doctor and nurse that contracted the disease, and they are still alive 20 years later.

A FATHERS ANGUISH

He wanted to know what could be done to save his daughter

In the late 1980s I took care of a thirty-three year old woman who was suffering from late stage A.I.D.s. At that time, we had nothing in the way of treatment for that disease. It seems that this woman was an I.V. drug abuser and she probably contracted the disease from sharing needles. Many I.V. drug abusers contracted A.I.D.s this way.

The only person who visited this patient was her father; no mother, brothers, sisters or friends came to see her. The father visited everyday in the late afternoon. The patient was very restless and diaphoretic. Her speech was inarticulate. She was unable to accept any food or drink and her only hydration came from I.V. fluid.

One day wanting to speak to me the father approached the nurse's station. One could see the anguish in his eyes. Looking in his eyes I it looked as if he was pleading with me. He wanted to know what could be done to save his daughter. I explained there was nothing we could do to cure her. The best we could do was to keep her comfortable.

I told him that when she died I would inform the doctor and ask him if he wanted to pronounce or he wanted me to pronounce (in Florida a nurse may pronounce in the hospital). Then I would inform him of his daughter's expiration. Next, he asked me how I would know she was dead. I explained once she no longer is breathing and no longer has a pulse or blood pressure, I would call the doctor and him, and let him know she has passed. Lucky for me when she died I was not on duty, so I did not have to make those calls.

YOU'RE GOLDEN IN 30 DAYS
All were operated on by the same doctor

There are good doctors, and there are bad doctors, there are doctor families, where sons and daughters follow in their father's footsteps. Not all relatives of doctors inherit the abilities of their parents, but they try. The problem with trying, is that if they stink at what they do, they may hurt a lot of people along the way. The patients keep coming, because they have no idea how many bad outcomes were produced by the relative who takes too long to do a procedure their father could do in one third the time. There are numbers kept for bad surgical outcomes, that is, a death in the first 30 days after surgery. Of course, the death must be related to the surgery, like infection, sepsis, heart failure, surgical misadventure (a screw up) and other causes. Doctors take extraordinary efforts to have patients stay alive until the 31st day, then they don't really give a shit what happens. This is a story about one of those physicians, the son of a well known heart surgeon that followed in his father's footsteps.

I was working for an agency at the time, and working for an agency, you are sent to different hospitals, and do not know where you will be working in the hospital until you get there. Hospitals use agency people as a last resort because they cost more. You show up to the nursing office, and they assign you to the place where you will work the shift. I had been working for this particular agency almost two years, and they had me assigned to the same hospital for those two years. On this night, I was assigned to a surgical intensive care unit to replace a nurse that was assigned to care for a group of patients on ventilators. When I got to the unit, I saw that there was a row of patients post op on ventilators. There must have been at least twelve or so, and I was told there were so many that the hospital had to rent additional units. All the patients were separated by a curtain around each one, and all were operated on by the same doctor.

I had never seen anything like this before, so when I had the chance, I asked the other nurses "what the hell is going on." They were disgusted, and told me that all of the patients had underwent open heart surgery at the hands of this one doctor. They then told me about the 30 day rule, and related that this pile of patients was the largest group he had ever screwed up. Usually they could handle the messes without using agency staff to fill in. I couldn't believe what I was hearing, I had seen doctors make a mess, but this was ridiculous, unbelievable.

Throughout the evening families of the patients came and went, until this one family showed up to see their father. The father had been kept alive by the ventilator for two weeks or so, and they had had enough. They were armed with a medical power of attorney, and told the nurse that they wanted the ventilator turned off. They had evidentially been reading quite a bit about the father's current condition and were armed with considerable knowledge that routine families didn't have. They wanted the machine disconnected and the breathing tube pulled out, and if their father could not breathe on his own, they wanted him to die a natural death. They were tired of watching him lie there being kept alive artificially. The nurse reported that she had to call the doctor and tell him their wishes, and they agreed. The doctor took the call at home, and told the nurse that he was on the way to the hospital and not to disconnect anything until he arrived, and he would do it.

Well, the doctor came running into the unit all out of breath to confront the family. Remember, the patient was in the window where the death would be charged against the doctor. He heard the families request and began to preach against it. He tried everything he could think of to dissuade the family from disconnecting the patient, all to no avail. I was in the room next to the alcove where the family surrounded the patient, so I heard everything they all said. The family persisted with their wish to unplug the ventilator regardless of the doctor's pleas. Finally, I heard the doctor resort to something so bad that I couldn't believe my ears. He said "you're not giving him a chance to live, you're just wanting to kill your father, this is nothing short of murder." I wanted to run around the corner and punch him in the mouth. I couldn't imagine that rotten bastard saying that to a family. The family took it very quietly, and again told the doctor that they would not leave until they saw this through, and they wanted the ventilator disconnected right now. The doctor threw up his hands and shouted "very well" as he stormed out cursing to himself. The RN pulled the breathing tube and shut the machine down, and the patient died on the spot. The family said their goodbyes and left, but before they did, they were surrounded by a group of RN's who told them that they did the right thing. I'm glad I got the chance to tell someone this story, it needed to be told, for that family.

TALK ABOUT A JOKE!

A longstanding policy of the inmates running the insane asylum

Nurses aides are a scarce commodity, at least in the hospitals I worked in. At the most, you would get one per wing of the hospital, and most of the time there were none. Occasionally, a school teaching people to become aides would bring a class to the floor of a hospital to let them get some experience, and practice the skills the students were taught in class. Being a male nurse, I never saw an aide on the telemetry floor, they sometimes came in the class, but I never saw one, and assumed that they were helping nurses at the other end of the hallway.

On this particular day a class was on the floor somewhere, when I received an admission to one of the empty rooms I was covering. I went into the room and deposited a packet of all the free things provided by the hospital to the new patients. These were toothpaste, a toothbrush, soap, towel wash cloth etc. I turned down the bed, and checked the bathroom to make sure everything was clean and ready before the patient arrived. (these were some of the things an aide would do) As I finished, down the hall came the female patient in a wheelchair, pushed by a volunteer. I welcomed her, and asked if she could change into a hospital gown by herself, and she said she could, so I asked her to do that.

When she finished, I picked up her clothes from the bed to hang them in the closet for her. The closets in each room were double sliding door affairs next to each other, providing considerable space for storing things for each patient. I slid aside one door for this patient's clothes, and staring me in the face was two black nurse's aides from the class assigned to our unit. I reached past one of them and retrieved a hanger and hung the patient's clothes on the clothing bar. I said nothing to the two aides, and slid the door back shut enclosing them back in the closet, and I left the room. About five minutes later the two students came quietly out of the room, and slithered away down the hallway. Now I know why I never saw them working on the floor.

THE NEW JOB
The whole thing was a waste of time

I saw an ad for a nursing instructor placed by a school that taught nursing assistants. I submitted an application on-line and was accepted to teach in the classroom. Something seemed amiss from the start. I found out that the school was essentially paid for by the federal government. It was a private affair, but 100% of the revenue was from government programs trying to get welfare recipients into the workplace. The government provided childcare and tuition, plus a stipend to any and all welfare recipients that applied to the school. Unknown to me at the time, both the school and the students were working the scam to the hilt. The welfare mothers in the class got free child care which gave them free time to commiserate with their friends during class, and to play on their phones all day. They were not there to learn anything, nor where they there to become nurse's aides, they were there to game the system. The school was there to game the system on their end by providing a sham education, issue worthless certificates, and produce nothing of value into the workplace.

There were two nurses working the classroom program which called for four nurses at the minimum. The two were distraught trying to keep the place going night and day without relief, they were fried. They were so happy to see me come aboard because the last hire lasted half of one class and quit, which gave them no relief. I had a week of orientation to go through rotating through classrooms, labs, and administration to learn paperwork. During my lab orientation I got to talk to the lab instructor who immediately cautioned me. She told me not to argue with any student over anything, just either ignore them, or give them their way. She said, I would only cause myself grief, because the school would not expel or discipline any student because the federal money for that student would stop if they quit. So, the message was to keep the students attending regardless of their behavior no matter how troublesome they became. In short, the welfare mothers did what they wanted to do, and shouted out anything they felt like with no repercussions to them. Hell of a way to run the school, oops, I meant scam. The next day I participated in an awards program for a class moving into the next cycle in their program. There were nine cycles, and a student could be enrolled into any cycle, as long as they finished all nine, they would graduate. In this ceremony, there were boxes of little pins (the type you would put on a hat) and one by one the students names were called, and they received any number of these pins for things they accomplished, like washing their hands, wearing a hair net, farting, etc. The welfare mothers strutted and did a little dance after each received their pins. I immediately thought of the football players doing the same type dances after they scored a touchdown. The whole thing was a waste of time, but I didn't fully realize it at the time.

After a week goofing off, I was to teach my first class. I took my time making up a killer class for the students, it was an introduction to the circulatory and respiratory systems. I made a syllabus with lecture, and visual aids with x-ray slides it was going to kick off my new teaching career with a bang.

The class filed into the room, and I got a look at the mix of students. They were a mix of black and Latin American young people. I introduced myself and began the lecture. I'm a talker, so explaining things clearly is one of the things I'm good at. I noticed about a third of the class were interested and taking notes (these were the students attending their first class in the first module) and the rest were just sitting there looking bored. After the first half hour, a welfare mother raised her hand with a question. She asked "where is the movie" I said "there is no movie, this is a lecture where you are taught subject matter." She then said "we always have a movie" and several of her friends nodded in agreement. I smelled trouble brewing right away. The troublemaker persisted with furthering her argument with her three friends joining in with their own verbal arguments. At this point the class became a free for all with much of the class telling them to shut up and let me teach the class.

I realized immediately that there had been a long standing policy of the inmates running the insane asylum, and I don't subscribe to that bullshit. I decided on the spot that this was not an environment I could function under, and put the class on hold. I went to the locker room and told the full time instructor I was replacing, that I was leaving the school and would not be back. I walked past the classroom and left through a side door to the parking lot, got in my car in full view of the class, and drove away. (incidentally, my car was the oldest in the parking lot, as all the welfare mothers were driving new cars, and two of their cars were black Jaguars). The school was back where they started a week before with only two instructors, and I was richer by a week's pay for attending orientation.

I CAN FLY, I CAN FLY

There was nothing he could do to avoid the collision

If one nurse on a unit gets caught-up in their work, they usually ask others if they need any help. This was the case working on a unit that received cases brought in by helicopter. I was through passing my food trays and had given all my meds as my patient load was not as heavy as usual. Just like any other experience, you get a break once in a while. I picked out the nurse working next to me and asked her if I could help her. She told me that the patient in the private room needed to be fed.

I went into the room and the tray was already on the over the bed table. I removed the cover and cut up the meat for the patient. He was sitting in the bed ready to be fed. He had both arms in casts with a bar going from the elbow to the rest of the cast around his torso, he was a mess. He was a typical motorcycle gang member with the raggedy pony tail, teeth missing, and tattoos all over. His age was about 55 and he was very thin. He also had "road rash" on his face due to contact with the road during the accident. (this is typical of motorcycle accidents where the rider scrapes or rolls along the highway leaving his skin behind) I have seen scraping so bad that all the flesh was gone, and even the bone was worn away especially on the hands because the victim always puts his hands out as a reflex trying to stop himself.

This fellow was eager to eat and gobbled everything down in short order, he seemed to be very hungry. When he finished the plate, I held up the liquids for him to drink through a straw. It was at that point that I was able to ask him what had happened to him. He told me that he was tooling along on the interstate doing the speed limit of 70 MPH. He was relaxing with his feet up enjoying the ride without a worry in the world. The sun was shining and the motorcycle was performing very well. The interstate has three lanes in each direction with a wide median separating the north and south bound lanes. The median has both trees and heavy untrimmed brush throughout its length.

The motorcyclist heard the crashing of cars and screeching of tires in the opposing lanes, with a cloud of dirt, steam, and smoke rising above the tall brush in the median. Continuing along unimpeded he was still doing fine tooling along. Suddenly crashing through the brush came a silver car careening toward him in reverse. The car continued to clear the brush, and came flying across the shoulder of the road to his right, and proceeded to cross in front of him backwards. It was directly in his path and he saw that he was going to hit the car just behind the rear wheel. There was nothing he could do to avoid the collision especially travelling at 70 MPH. He struck the vehicle and was launched into the air passing over the trunk of the car and continuing to fly through the air unimpeded. He was thinking at the time "this isn't so bad my body missed smashing into the car." He then realized that he was going to land while still travelling at very close to 70 MPH. Coming down head first he put his hands and arms out to break his fall. He contacted the highway and witnessed his arms breaking as he began to skid along until he folded up and started to tumble down the road landing in a heap of broken bones and bloody flesh. He laid there for a minute or so assessing the situation and feeling no immediate pain. He told me that he got a feeling of well being which left quickly when the pain began. He reported that he began screaming, and didn't stop until he got to the emergency room and was sedated. He had been in a couple small accidents before, but this one made him rethink the motorcycle lifestyle. The accident was not his fault, but he was the only one hurt in the damage on his side of the highway, the people in the car were fine.

NEW SHOES

He told me he was keeping the trike

The next accident happened at an intersection and involved one vehicle, a three wheeled motorcycle. The owner of the motorcycle went for a ride to purchase a new pair of leather shoes. He owned a car, but it was a nice sunny day so he decided to take the motorcycle. After selecting his new shoes, he decided to wear them home, and place his old ones in a saddle bag on the bike. Driving home, he came to a red light and braked, but the shiny new leather on the sole of his new shoe slipped off the brake pedal and onto the gas. Caught by surprise, he rocketed through the intersection and sideswiped a no parking sign on the opposing curb line. Since he was sitting with both legs exposed, when he sideswiped the pole, it caught the inside of his knee forcing his leg out to the side. The motorcycle continued past the pole, forcing his leg so far to the outside it separated it at the hip joint and fell onto the street. The motorcycle continued down the street leaving the entire leg on the sidewalk. Eventually the bike came to a halt and the poor rider was brought into the hospital minus a leg which could not be reattached. He came to me post op where he was closed at the hip, and did quite well on crutches. He told me that he was keeping the trike because he built it himself, and learned that he couldn't ride it with new shoe on. Notice I said shoe, not shoes.

HIT AND RUN
He was operated on and a pin was inserted

Most Americans have health insurance through their employers. If they loose employment they loose their health insurance and become medically indigent. Very few Americans can afford to be hospitalized without health insurance. When working as a home health care coordinator I had to setup services for one such patient.

The patient in question was a forty year old male machinist. Upon returning home from work, he discovered his house was being burglarized. The burglar being discovered fled. Instead of calling police, the home owner chased the thief down the road. The burglar jumped in his car, which was parked down the street from the house he was robbing. While attempting to get away the thief hit the home owner with the car. The hit and run resulted in a right leg fracture for the victim. Lucky for him a neighbor saw him being hit by the car and called 9/11. The ambulance arrived and took him to a nearby hospital. There he was operated on and a pin was inserted into his leg. The doctor who performed the operation told the patient he could not return to work for at least a month. According to the patient, the day he was discharged from the hospital his incision site started to drain. He told the discharging doctor about the drainage. The discharging doctor assured him that it was nothing to worry about.

Once he got home, he called his employer and informed him he could not return to work for at least a month. This resulted in his termination and loss of insurance (he had Blue Cross). A week later drainage had become worse and he also developed a fever, so he came to my hospital, which was twenty-two miles from his home. He was admitted through the E.R. and sent to surgery where he has his wound drained and a wound vac applied. He was then transferred to the orthopedic floor where he was given I.V. antibiotics. After three days on the orthopedic floor, it was decided that he could be discharged home on a wound vac. When I arrived on the floor, I explained that to rent a wound vac for two weeks would cost $5,000.00 and a nurse would have to come out at least six times to change the dressing and that would cost $900.00.

This is when the patient told me his story. He told me due to the loss of his job and insurance he could not afford the wound vac and home health care nurses. Next, I did something I had never done before. I called up the company I used for wound vacs and requested they provide this patient with a free machine. I explained the patient's situation to the company representative. I reminded her of all the business I gave her, and I could give that business to another company. She agreed to give the patient a free wound vac. The hospital agreed to pay for his home nursing because it was cheaper to have his care done at home than in the hospital. The next day the patient I told the patient he was getting a free wound vac and six free nursing visits. The patient was ecstatic; not only was he getting a free wound vac and free nursing visits, but just before I arrived a police detective showed up and informed the patient the burglar had been captured. Because he lost his insurance, if I did not become his advocate, he probably would have been sent home on wet to dry dressings. The floor nurses would have shown him how to change his dressing and gave him some supplies (not enough to last two weeks). If he went home on wet to dry dressings there would have been a good chance he would have returned to the hospital with another abscess. The reason why I pulled some strings for him was he seemed like a decent guy who had some bad luck. The vac must have worked, he never returned to the hospital.

STOMP HARDER ON THE GAS
A Florida State Trooper walked onto the floor

Some Hospitals have medical office buildings alongside them, or across the street. In this case, the medical offices were partially joined to the hospital by a glass walkway so patients needing x-rays or blood work could traverse between sites. Alongside the medical office building was a parking lot situated so that patients could enter he offices by several means. They could walk around the front of the building, or they could walk to the end of the parking lot and go up a group of low wide stairs and enter the glass walkway through a glass door. On this day, a gomer (a gomer is an elderly person generally suffering from some form of dementia) in a big Cadillac (gomers like big cars, the bigger the better) was parking in the parking lot in a space facing the glass walkway. From his position he could look out the windshield of the car, and watch people passing through the walkway. Somehow, the driver stomped on the gas pedal thinking he was braking and launched the big Cadillac up the staircase and crashed through the glass walkway. At the same time some doctor's patient was laboring past on crutches with a cast on his leg.

The big Cadillac struck the poor guy on crutches and broke both of his legs, coming to rest in the walkway. A rescue squad was called and the unfortunate man was deposited in the emergency department to be treated. The driver of the car reported that he didn't know what had happened and tried to blame the accident on any number of things beyond his control. In order to get at the root of the problem, he was admitted to the hospital to be worked up for a series of tests related to TIA. (transient ischemic attack, or unexplained period of unconsciousness)

The driver was admitted to a room at the end of the hallway on the floor where I was assigned. He was an overweight, overbearing, rubber faced blow bag on first observation. One of those guys that feels he is in charge of everything, and you had better listen to him or else. He was running the nurses around using a very demanding tone, and was quickly becoming the most annoying asshole you ever met.

The second day after his admission, the elevator door opened, and a Florida State Trooper walked onto the floor. He went over to the desk and asked for the blow bag. He was directed down to the end of the hall where the room was located. He entered the room, and remained there for about five minutes, asking the blow bag to see his drivers license. Blow bag retrieved his wallet from the bedside table and gave his license to the State Trooper. The trooper then explained that he had been sent to the hospital to take the license into his possession, and inform the driver that he would not be able to drive in the State of Florida again. The blow bag had been involved in a crash two months before, where he crashed into a house almost killing the woman inside. The gomer had done serious injury and damage in two separate accidents. His license was revoked permanently, causing him to scream at the top of his lungs that he would sue the trooper, and the State of Florida. He further states that everyone involved would hear from his lawyer. The trooper was long gone in the elevator and he was still screaming at the top of his lungs. We later found out that he had gotten his Cadillac out of the shop two days before this accident, and it was towed right back to the same shop to be fixed again. The blow bag was discharged that evening, I never found out how the poor guy with the broken legs made out.

There are not many books on the market dealing with nursing or nursing cases. The word gomer was coined by another author in his stories about gomers in the emergency room at the hospital where he was working. In order to understand why the elderly are called gomers you should know what emergency room staff are confronted with on a daily basis.

Once a gomer gets it in his or her head that visiting the

ER (emergency room of a hospital) will get them attention in a very short time, they make a habit of it. They become what nurses call FREQUENT FLIERS, who visit for some mundane matters feeling the ER is the answer for everything. Examples are, "I haven't had a BM (bowel movement) today", or "I ate something spicy and my stomach is upset", or "my neighbor said I looked flushed." If they went to the doctor's office, they would sit in the waiting room all day and when they got to see the doctor, they would be sent home with a sample of some useless medication just to get rid of them because 90% of the time there is nothing wrong with them.

Most gomers have a driver's license and only drive in good weather and during the day time. They are terrible drivers, and often go up any on ramp they see, and wind up in another state or city. They are also found in a store parking lot walking around looking for their car. If you ask them what color the car is, or the make, they can't tell you, but they say "I'll know it when I see it."

It is important to understand that you can't talk rationally to an irrational person. Irrational people will never understand a rational argument no matter how long you try and phrase it correctly for them. You are wasting your time talking to them, so you have to find a way to (turf them) get someone in another area to deal with them.

When they are admitted to the hospital for observation, they become a nightmare for the floor nurse, who is at the end of the road of turfing. The floor nurse gets all the turfed patients from every other department of the hospital including outpatient. Gomers admitted to the floor are a hell of a source of money for everyone that sees them. Amazingly, gomers love tests. They love talking to the staff they meet in the hospital because at home they hardly get any company. In many cases they only hear from sons and daughters when they want something from them. Gomers feel that eventually after all the tests, they will have all their ills resolved and be able to function like they could when they were younger. What they don't understand, and never will understand is that they are the dairy cow of the hospital and doctors. Eventually, they will be discharged back to wherever they came from, and the gomer cycle will be repeated time and time again. They have no idea that they have just bought a new Mercedes for the doctor (thank you very much) or a new mansion for the hospital system chief executive officer. (again, thank you very much).

NO FOOD FOR YOU 6 MONTHS
There was a large plastic bag taped to her neck

Working 3-11 shift for an agency I was assigned to a row of five rooms containing patients who were expected to be in the hospital for a long time, or had been in the hospital for a long time. Large hospital systems provide their own employees with medical insurance rather than dealing with medical insurance firms. It is much cheaper to handle everything in-house for less cost to the hospital. This effectively removes the profit a medical insurance company would make, and transfers it to the hospitals bottom line instead.

So, when something goes wrong with a person covered by the hospitals coverage that requires long term care, instead of putting that person into a long-term care situation in a nursing home, the hospital keeps a row of rooms in the building to house them in-house and hires a nurse to see to their daily care and feeding. The bulk of these patients are incapacitated in one way or another. The incapacitation can be either mentally or physically such as a stroke, or a problem like I describe below.

Of the five patients I was assigned one in particular stood out causing me to never put her memory aside with many others. My first encounter was at the beginning of the shift when I went into each room to see what I was confronting for the shift. Here was an alert and oriented woman about fifty years old in very good physical condition. She had one major problem, there was a large plastic bag taped to the side of her neck on the left side. The bag was somewhat opaque, but I could see bubbles of what looked like saliva foaming in the one third filled bag. There was also an abdominal feed tube poking out of her abdomen which meant she received cans of nutrient at regular intervals throughout the day.

I talked to her briefly introducing myself and doing my vital signs and my examination moving quickly through the chores to get to the rest of the patients. You tabulate as you go, making mental notes of what to tackle first, and what to leave to later. I went to the next room which was a turn and baste case. (turning the patient to a different position blocked up by pillows every two hours to preserve their skin from ulcers) Turn and baste cases are sad cases because they are not alert and cannot say or do anything for themselves. If you neglect these cases, they become nightmares in one day, because their skin rots away on their bodies exposing them to massive sores and infections. You must turn them on a schedule regardless of the needs of other patients in your care. I preferred to turn them more frequently because they were not going to catch me not doing my job, I would do my job and a little extra.

The next patient was paralyzed from the chest down and in an air bed so turning and basting was not necessary. The bed was like a sand box of plastic beads that flow like water. There is an air agitation system that bubbles up air from the bottom making the plastic beads bubble under the patient. The patient could not develop sores while on the bed. This patient was not alert or oriented either, just lying on the bed with a large bag of Hyperalimentation hanging (food and fats in a bag continuously infused through an IV placed under the collar bone. I pulled back the covers and found that his feet were a mess. His nails were terribly long, and between his toes was the biggest mess of dead skin, lint, and all kinds of gook I had ever seen. I resolved to make that one of my projects, cleaning his feet up so they looked somewhat normal. No one had done that in about six months or more. The rest to the patients were unremarkable cases well within my scope of care, none were connected to heart monitors.

First, I tackled the turn and base patient who needed a haircut badly, his hair was the worst rats nest of tangled wool I had ever seen. I moved him to his back and sat the bed up into a sitting position and raised the whole bed up to my level. I had a pair of bandage scissors in my pocket so I pulled them out and went to work on the wool. I got a comb from the supplies machine and used it to see what things looked like after the wool was cut away. Eventually he started to look like a human, and when his head was washed and his hair combed, he looked great. I was changing the bed when the social worker stopped in to visually check on the patient. She seemed astounded and asked me if the barber had been to see the patient. I held up the bandage scissors and she got the idea, she was impressed.

I moved to the feet job taking a basin of hot soapy water with me. I wet his feet and started grabbing the gunk with the wash cloth and rinsing it in the water. I had completed one foot and had to get new water, the smell and sight of what was coming out from between his toes was making me sick. I dumped the load, refreshed the basin and accomplish the work on the other foot taking care to thoroughly drying between each toe as there was brand new red skin under the mess and I didn't want to leave it wet. When I finished the washing, I gave him a nail clip and moved on to the bag lady.

To my surprise she was trained and capable of dumping the cans of nutrient into the feed bag herself, so that saved me a few minutes. I asked her what jobs I could perform for her, and did she want anything I could fetch for her. She said she was OK and needed nothing, she did ask me if I could stay for a few minutes and talk. I took a seat and she began immediately relating how she came to be in this position sitting in bed with the bag on her neck and the feed tube. She related that she was having some gastric reflux (stomach acid bubbling up into the esophagus) and the doctor wanted to scope her to investigate it. She was also having thick or hard types of food getting stuck at the valve into the stomach. She walked into the hospital with two minor problems expecting to be home by lunch, that was not going to be the case. She was prepped and put to sleep for the procedure, the doctor passed the scope down her esophagus to examine her issues. He saw a narrowing of the esophagus where it enters her stomach, so he inflated the cuff on the scope to stretch the constriction. Whatever happened after that in the exam room the doctor forgot to deflate the cuff and pulled the scope out of her mouth. Attached to the scope was her esophagus that had been ripped out by the inflated cuff. It had severed the esophagus at the entrance to the stomach. She was rushed immediately to the operating room where a repair to the esophagus was done and a feeding tube was inserted into the stomach.

To prevent her from swallowing, a hole was made in the side of her neck and a tube put into her esophagus to prevent anything from passing down the esophagus until it was healed. That accounted for the bag of spit. The biggest problem was why she was admitted long term to the hospital, the esophagus has an extremely small blood supply, it is a tube not an organ. Healing takes months when the entire esophagus is torn apart because you need lots of blood to heal something. Once the esophagus is healed, she was facing all the additional surgeries to repair her neck and abdomen. And remember she walked into the hospital with a few minor problems she could have lived the rest of her life with. Ask me why I don't have a Colonoscopy.

DAY TRIPPING

They gave the keys to the van to one of the patients

One good thing about nursing is, you can always find a part-time job. Hospitals are open 24/7, so they are always happy to have a nurse who wants to work only weekends or nights. One of the many part-time jobs I had, was at a long term private psych hospital. Even though I had limited psych experience, (psychiatric nursing class in college) they were happy to have someone with the initials R.N. after their name, who wanted to work weekends only.

Some of their patients had been there over twenty years. You can imagine, being forced to live in a facility 24/7 could be very hard, so patients who the psychiatrists deemed appropriate were allowed to go out on day trips. The trips were to the beach, stores, restaurants, or parks. The patients (four to six at a time) traveled to their destination in an unmarked hospital van accompanied by two staff members.

Two of the day trips were very memorable. The first involved a young woman in her early twenties, who was a ward of the State of New Jersey. She was a patient at our facility because we had one of the only programs in the country for deaf psychiatric patients. This woman could easily become angry and get very violent. Even though she was small, she was very strong. One day during one of her episodes, she picked up a T.V. and threw it across the room mashing it against a wall. Although she was prone to violence, she never gave me any problems, for some reason she liked me. That is one thing about psychiatric patients, for no rational reason they may like one staff member and dislike another, but if they were rational, they would not be institutionalized.

After behaving herself for several weeks, the doctors decided this young lady could go on a day trip. I did not go on the trip, but I heard about it when they group returned. The young women, and three other patients, along with two psych tech (psych techs are like nurse's aides) went to Walmart. The woman had a breakdown in Walmart. The two techs got her out of the store along with the other patients and back to the van. Since it took both techs to control the young woman, they gave the keys of the van to one of the other patients, so he could drive the van back to the hospital. Somehow the psych patient managed to get the van back to the hospital without incident.

DAY TRIPPER

He yelled at the top of his lungs

The second memorable day trip involved going to the beach on Labor Day. The main character in this trip was a man in his late twenties. This young man had a father who was a retired high-ranking naval officer. When the young man turned eighteen, he decided to join the Marine Corps. During basic training he had a seizure, which resulted in his discharge from the Marine Corps. After six months had passed, he joined the Army. He did not tell the Army that he had a seizure, or that he had been in the Marines. He managed to get through both basic and medic training in the Army without a seizure. Following his training, he was stationed at an Army hospital. The hospital soon discovered their Dilantin supply was being depleted illegally. (Dilantin is a drug used to control seizures).

The hospital tracked the missing drug to the medic, and they also discovered he had been in the Marines. As a result, he was discharged from the Army. Besides having seizures, he also had psychiatric problems, so he ended up in our facility.

The doctors decided he could go on a day trip to the beach planned for Labor Day. This young man and five other patients boarded the hospital van for the beach. Upon arriving, it was discovered the beach was packed. Getting out of the van, the man yelled at the top of his lungs, "we are psych patients out on a day trip." People either vacated the beach or moved to the extreme ends of the beach. It was funny because the six psych patients had a large expanses of beach to themselves.

JESUS

Jesus ran into the wall

While on the neuro floor of a large community hospital I met Jesus Christ. Jesus Christ was a twenty something white male with long blonde hair that came down to the middle of his back. Jesus was arrest by the local police for trespass. While at the county jail he told the other prisoners that he was Jesus Christ. One the prisoners responded that "if you are truly Jesus Christ run into the wall head first and the angels will prevent you from hitting the wall." Jesus ran into the wall head first and the angels did not prevent the crash, they also did not prevent the head laceration he received. (remember, everyone involved here was a blithering idiot) He was taken to the emergency room via ambulance, and because there was no room on the psychiatric unit he was sent to neurology. This was not unusual, in fact the nurses used to joke about it, we called the neurology unit psych over-flow.

In the middle of the night, Jesus Christ got out of his bed stark naked and walked into a semi-private room housing two fifty year old women, and started to preach to them. Luckily the women had a sense of humor laughed, and took it with a grain of salt. The next day Jesus was moved to the psych unit. There, this Jesus Christ met another patient who claimed he was Jesus Christ. I was told later, by one of the psych nurses, that the two Jesus Christs used to challenge each other in quoting scripture, to prove who was the real Jesus Christ. The issue was never resolved to either's satisfaction.

DRUNKS

There are basically two kinds of drunks

One Saturday evening I was floated to the ER. Floating is fairly common. If your unit is over staffed, and another unit is understaffed, someone from your unit will be sent to the understaffed unit that's what is called floating. On weekend nights in the ER, you tend to get car accidents, drug overdoses, the losers of bar fights, shooting and stabbing victims, and drunks. When I was a boy growing up in the 1960's public drunkenness was a crime, the police did not take you to the emergency room, instead you went to jail. Today, at least in my part of Florida, law enforcement brings you to the ER. Unfortunately, in the past someone died in the drunk tank from lack of medical care, so things have changed.

There are basically two kinds of drunks; the belligerent and the friendly. The belligerent wants to hit you and does not follow directions. The belligerent drunk also likes to take off his/her clothes. An example of a belligerent drunk was a female, in her late twenties, who the police dropped off in the ER. The woman was not only drunk, but had been in a bar fight. She was put in one of the exam rooms, where a female nurse took her vital signs and tended to her wounds. When the nurse who was attending to her left the room, the drunk took off all her clothes and walked stark naked into the ER waiting room. Her nurse went after her and tried to get her back into the exam room. The drunk refused to go back and kicked her in the stomach. A code gray was called (a code gray means we have a violent patient) the evening maintenance man and myself were able to get the woman back into her exam room and apply leather restraints.

The friendly drunk, does not want to fight, and everybody he meets is his friend. I was lucky this drunk was friendly. A family member of one of the ER patients informed the triage nurse (the nurse in the ER who decides the priority in which patients are seen) that he saw a man lying face down where the ambulances park. The triage nurse informed me of the situation. I and a nurse's aide went to investigate. Sure enough, there was what appeared to be a tall black man lying face down in the parking lot. We managed to get him on a stretcher and bring him into one of the ER's exam rooms. The man smelled of alcohol. I asked the man if he was sick or drunk, he responded "drunk." I next informed him that he was in a hospital and asked him if he would like to see a doctor. He said "no." I asked him his name and he gave me his first name Ray, but would not give me a last name. I checked his pockets for ID and the only thing I found was one dollar. I called the charge nurse and informed him of the situation. The charge nurse asked Ray his last name and address and Ray refused to answer. The charge nurse told me to stay with Ray and he was going to call the police. Ray asked me why the police were called, he stated "I did not steal anything." I said "I know you did not steal anything Ray, but what are we supposed to do? We find you face down in the parking lot, you do not want to see a doctor, and you will not give us your last name or address." Ray then started to laugh and playful slapped me in the face, and told me "you're a bad nigger." I responded "Ray you are not only drunk, but you are color blind too."

Next Ray told me he had to go to urinate. I put Ray in a wheelchair and wheeled him into the bathroom, I am 5'9" and Ray was at least 6'2". Ray was leaning on me while he was urinating in the toilet. I managed to get him back in the wheelchair and waiting outside the bathroom were two policemen. The officer asked Ray is last name and Ray responded "I am a roofer, I am a good roofer, I do your roof, you call Jones Roofing." The officer told Ray it was 10 o'clock on Saturday night he did not think anybody was at Jones Roofing. The officer then asked Ray for his address.

Ray answered "Myrtle Ave." The officer said "Ray I need a street number. What am I supposed to do, drop you off on somebody's front lawn"? Finally, Ray gave the officer a street address and I helped Ray into the police car. I thought to myself that night, the police were Ray's taxi service home, and the taxpayer is footing the bill.

I'LL TAKE TWO UNITS PLEASE
She had just flown in from California a few hours before

I was working the evening shift in a major trauma center, when I was given an admission into one of my rooms under exceptionally different circumstances. Usually an admission is sent up to the floor for a stay ranging from one night to indefinite. In this case the admission was for just several hours, and the patient was to be discharged that evening. She was walking into the room, and getting up and walking out. During her admission I was to administer two units of packed red blood cells. (in other words, she was getting two pints of blood) The voluminous paperwork usually done by the nurse on an admission was not present, it was just a manila folder with several sheets of paper in it, which was a great relief to me. The patient was escorted to the room by someone from admitting, and she was placed onto the bed fully clothed except she took off her shoes. Of course, this was really unusual, but considering that she was going home after I administered the blood, I played along and said nothing. I went into the folder and there was a doctor's order for the two units of packed cells, so I called the blood bank to see if they were ready to be picked up. After checking their inventory, the blood bank reported that they had the two units ready, Type and Cross was completed and I could pick up the first unit at the blood bank.

I should note, that type and cross consists of making sure that the patients blood type and the donors type are both the same or compatible. Cross means crossmatching the blood for antibodies. Most of the population in this country have similar or the same antibodies that they have built up over their lifetime from contracting the same type illnesses. The real problem with crossmatching is when an immigrant from a distant country brings different antibodies into their blood. These antibodies have to be matched to administer blood to that person, and sometimes those antibodies are difficult to get. Additionally, when an individual receives an inordinate amount of blood transfusions they may have trouble making crossmatches because of the varied donors.

I retrieved the administration tubing and the unit of blood from the blood bank, and set it up on an IV pole at the bedside. I had another RN verify both the patient and the unit of blood with me and I began the first transfusion. You are required to stay with the patient for the first part of the transfusion because if the patient has a reaction to the transfusion you will be present to stop the blood flow and call the doctor and report the problem. While I was waiting, I began asking the patient if she lived near the hospital. She reported that she had just flown in from California a few hours before, and came from the airport to the hospital. I thought this was very unusual, but everything about this case was unusual up to this point. The transfusion was doing well, so I left to tend to other patients, returning at timed intervals to take vital signs as prescribed by protocol. Before the blood administration finished, I returned to the room and the patient told me that she had a daughter in the area, and she would be staying there. She further stated that her daughter had made all the arrangements for her to receive the blood upon her arrival in Florida. Again, I thought this was growing more and more unique.

The first unit of blood finished so I went to get the next unit from the blood bank. When I returned, I went through the same procedure as before with another RN and began administration of the next unit. While I was waiting in the room the patient began to disclose more information. She reported that she had an uncurable form of blood disorder that required frequent transfusions for her to live. She told me that several doctors in California had been ordering blood for her but when the total number of units reached well over a hundred units, they refused to continue ordering additional blood for her. Of course, this put her in a precarious position, so she told her daughter and the daughter secured a doctor here in Florida to order the blood for her. That was why she came directly to the hospital, and was leaving that night to go to her daughter's home. Since I was working in that hospital through an agency, I did not work that unit regularly and never saw the patient again. I did however wonder, how many units of blood were ordered for her here in Florida, and the ethical dilemma the doctors faced continuing to place that kind of burden on the hospitals blood supply. Obviously, this type of usage could not go on forever, just imagine what multiple patients of this type could do to the local blood bank.

SEE YOU ON THE WEEKEND
She could not get off work

I was not trained as a critical care RN or an ICU RN, however I was consistently asked to cover these areas in the hospitals where I worked. This particular shift was on a Tuesday afternoon. I had certifications in telemetry, and Advanced Cardiac Life Support, and both of these credentials were the same requirements as for nurses in critical care units. I was covering on an ICU unit that had a one nurse shortage for a particular shift. On these units the RN had a reduced number of patients because the acuity of the patient was higher. Some of the patients are unstable, and require a nurse to attend their needs full time with no time to see any other patients. On this particular day I received a post-op patient that had a life-threatening problem.

The patient had undergone surgery for cancer in her digestive tract. During surgery it was discovered that the cancer was far more extensive than originally thought, and the tissues were destroyed to the extent that the surgeon had nothing to sew to. He was unable to draw the tissues together because the sutures continued to tear through the remaining flesh. After numerous tries he could not continue, and closed the wound leaving the oozing tissue behind inside. The oozing collected in the digestive tract and after several hours the patient would develop the sensation of an impending bowel movement. When this happened, the patient needed a bed pan and would evacuate a quantity of red blood into the bed pan. Of course, this required the nurse to not only provide and empty and clean the bed pan, but to continuously provide fresh blood to the patient by way of a transfusion of whole blood. As you can imagine, this patient required full time care to keep her clean and to continue to get units of blood from the blood bank. We had to put it in as fast as it was running out.

The patient's condition was critical even though she was fully awake and able to assist with her bed pan needs throughout the shift. The woman could only stay alive with the constant administration of blood to replace that which she was losing into the bed pan. Since she was in Florida for the winter months only, she had no other kin in the state, and in fact her only daughter resided in New England. After the attempt to repair her digestive tract had failed, and there was no hope for recovery, the physician placed a call to the patient's daughter. Word had it that the physician had been able to make contact, and gave a full explanation of the patient's predicament to the daughter. It was explained to her that there was no hope for her mother and she would only remain alive with continuous transfusions, and even that was no guarantee that they would do the job. The daughter said that she fully understood the problem but she could not get off work until the weekend when she could fly to Florida to see her mother. I was told that the doctor could not believe what he was hearing, which required making an attempt to keep the mother alive until the weekend. This would require an almost unlimited supply of blood given over four days in an attempt to have the mother last until the daughter could get off work on Saturday.

The doctor returned to the patient's bedside, and I could see that he was utterly defeated. He explained the issue to the patient and informed her that he would write the orders to attempt to accomplish the almost impossible. I left the room during their conversation because I did not want to be exposed to the anguish in the room, and did not want any emotion to show during the tasks I had ahead of me for the rest of the shift. I continued to empty bed pans full of blood, and continued to administer another three units of blood until my shift was over. Over 60 units later the daughter arrived to see the mother.

WHO'S WRONG, ME OR HIM?
What medical school did you go to?

There are many safeguards present on a telemetry unit. There is always a monitor tech watching the screens connected to each patient's chest monitor. There are telemetry trained nurses present all the time, and there are code buttons in every room to be mashed if help is needed outside the unit staff.

A staff nurse walked up to me with an ECG strip that was given to her by the monitor tech. The tech noticed something she didn't like, and called the nurse over immediately. The nurse searched me out on the next wing because her tele skills were not great and she had never seen the heart rhythm before. I had never seen the rhythm before except in classes, it was third degree heart block. This was a rhythm incompatible with life. A patient in this rhythm could not last long if they remained in this rhythm, it usually progresses into something immediately fatal.

I was walking toward the patient's room on the next wing when I passed the elevators and a door opened in front of me and it was the patient's cardiologist. I immediately showed the doctor the rhythm strip and told him that I had identified it as third-degree heart block. He looked at the strip and immediately looked back at me and with a sneer asked me what medical school I had graduated from (a snide attempt to illustrate that he was the doctor and I was not) I stuck to my guns and again said that it was indeed third degree block, and if he thought it wasn't then what rhythm did he want to call it. (he had a reason for denying my opinion which I would find out very quickly) He turned on his heel still carrying the strip and went immediately to the patients room. He was in the room less than a minute and proceeded to the fire tower across from the room and disappeared. I went to the room to see the patient after he exited, and the patient was sitting up in the bed alert. I asked her how she felt and she began to answer me when she went unconscious right in front of me. I immediately mashed the code button and began CPR on her until more help arrived. I also hit the intercom and had them page the cardiologist that had ducked into the fire tower. (He never answered the page) The code team worked on the woman for 15 minutes, and she was transferred to the CCU. She died there that night.

Now for the rest of the story that the cardiologist knew and I didn't until after the fact. The woman was admitted to the hospital for a Hysterectomy. While receiving her surgical work-up the cardiologist was summoned to clear the (the guy who came off the elevator) patient. She was a long time A-Fib (irregular heartbeat) patient, so while she was in the hospital the cardiologist wanted to take a stab at curing this problem with a different medication. He prescribed a medication new to the market called XXXXXXX. She was given the medication and after several doses she developed third degree heart block. The monitor tech picked it up, the nurse had the rhythm checked immediately, and action was being taken all within a couple minutes, when the doctor appeared and tried to quash the code which was in the process of being called. He knew immediately what was causing the third degree heart block and was in a panic. If he did the right thing he would have agreed with my call on the rhythm strip and called the code himself right away. Instead he ran from the scene making no timed notes in the chart, leaving nothing tangible to state that he had been there so he could claim later to the family that the cause of death was a heart attack, not his attempt to correct the A-Fib with the new medication. He knew he had caused the woman's death and refused to look me in the eye every time he came to the floor and we both knew why. Several weeks later I moved to home health to give it a try.

WHAT'S ONE LIFE

The physician advised me that everything was normal

While working at a local hospital I had the misfortune to work a shift on a telemetry unit one evening. It was unfortunate because a tragic event took place that absolutely could have been avoided. The scenario unfolds below.

I received an abdominal post-op patient from the recovery room and helped transfer her into the private room bed. She was middle aged, awake, alert, and able to move her arms and legs. Her vital signs were stable and she was talking to me. After placing her onto the bed I set about examining the wound and the surrounding area. There was a lividity mark on the lower portion of her side facing me. (lividity is a type of bruising that some post op patients have indicating blood has gotten into the tissues during surgery) In this case the procedure was to take a magic marker and mark the borders of the bruising, and watch it closely for any changes.

I reviewed the post op orders, and went to answer a light down the hallway. I returned to the post op room a little later and took another set of vital signs, and pulled back the covers to check her wound. The bruising on her side was unchanged. The patient reported feeling well and seemed to be doing fine. It is not every day that a patient has complications from surgery. Usually when the recovery room discharges a patient, they are very stable and out of any danger. I went back to doing my normal evening routine as a floor nurse.

Two hours later, I returned to the post-op patient's room and she was awake watching television but reported that she was not feeling as well as before, so I pulled back the covers and rechecked her wound. This time she had an extension of the bruising on her side, not a large change, but a change.

I marked the extension and retook her vital signs. There was a small decline in her blood pressure and a slight raise in her pulse rate. All were within normal limits so I resolved to watch her more closely. I began to return to the room more frequently, and recheck everything. As another hour approached, I made a decision to call the operating physician at home. He answered the phone, and I reported everything I had witnessed, including two advancements in bruising. The physician advised me that everything was normal, which I disputed. This was not my first merry-go-round with a post op patient. I wanted the physician to come in to see the patient, and possibly take her back to the OR because it looked to me like the patient was bleeding internally. It never hurts to be sure about something this serious. The doctor quickly became irate and told me not to call him again that evening.

I continued to monitor the patient, and everything continued to slide down hill, only she developed trapped air in her tissues called subcutaneous emphysema. I jumped on the phone again and called the doctor at home against his wishes. He was told everything I had experienced, but insisted that there was no reason to return to the hospital or to see the patient. Again, I challenged him and he became even more irate and hung up the phone on me.

At this point I was sure that I was right and the doctor was wrong, so I called the chief nursing officer on duty and asked him to come to the patient's room. In about five minutes he was in the room and I went over everything with him including showing him the five ever increasing magic marks I had made on her body all with the times written on each of them. At that point the patient announced "I'm going to die, aren't I" and I responded "not if I can help it." The nurse officer went to the phone and called the physician at home, and received the same rebuke I had received. He persisted as I had and he was also disconnected by the physician. He looked at me and shrugged his shoulders. I had don everything I was capable of doing and the only thing I could do at this point was to let the hospital wide nursing supervisor do his thing from this point forward. My shift had ended and I entered shift change, so I reported everything to the oncoming RN and went home.

When I returned the following evening to the same unit, I asked about the patient in the private room. The room was vacant but every nurse working knew the story by this time. I was told that the patient deteriorated throughout the night until 0530 when the physician came in and saw the patient. He was in a panic as he reviewed the nurses notes and vital signs throughout the night and called the family of the patient. By this time, she had virtually bled to death internally, so he asked the family to make her a no code. He gave the family some cock-a-mammie story and they bought it. If a code was called on the patient everyone else in the hospital would become aware of what he had done after reading the chart. The patient expired twenty minutes later and was taken to the morgue. The doctor went on his way whistling down the hallway and housekeeping was called to clean the room and prepare for the next patient.

Imagine what chance a nurse would have should she or he have called the family and told them the truth. In all probability the nurse would be black balled from working in the county, if they could ever work again. I knew a nurse who had taken a job working for a local heart doctor that specialized in heart catheterizations, she was a beautiful girl and was being courted by the married physician. They were so romantically involved that he began making promises to her that he could not keep. He also purchased things for her that should only be given to a spouse. Eventually, he promised to divorce his wife and marry her, which led to their downfall. In the end he got sued by the nurse, lost his family, coughed up $250,000.00 to the nurse and she had to sign a document that she would never work in the county again because his practice was there. Just imagine if she had been involved in a malpractice claim involving a patient death? She would have had to go to Nevada to get a job. Bad doctors are protected by everyone in their profession because they all have a vested interest in keeping things quiet. If every medical mistake became public knowledge, no one would go to a hospital or visit a doctor ever.

BED CLIMBERS, SHITTERS, AND SUNDOWNERS
Sometimes the patient can catch the nurse off guard

Did you ever wonder why all new cars look alike? When I was a kid we always were excited when the new cars were introduced into the showrooms. We used to go together to the dealership to look into the front window and marvel at what Detroit had provided. Those were the days when car guys built the cars. Today, new cars are designed and built by bean counters, and that's why they all look alike, and that's why instead of thirty different makes and models to choose from it is narrowed down to a few. Medicine has suffered the same fate as the beautiful cars we used to enjoy, it is run by bean counters. Today, certain diagnosis call for three days in a hospital, the money stops after the three days and the patient is sent home, well enough or not. Home health agencies lie on reports to extract as much money from each patient as they can. They milk each case for as much money as the insurance will pay for by falsifying reporting.

Doctors will string patients along promising that the third shot in the spine will do the trick, when they know the first shot will do the trick if they would put it in the right place. They have a chance to get the money for the three shots, so they hold back until the last visit to relieve the pain. They will only give you a prescription for 30 to 90 days to get the $300.00 office visit four times a year from the insurance.

Hospitals I know, looked for any reason to get rid of the older experienced nurses because a new group of nursing schools opened nearby, and now entry level nurses are cheap to hire. Hospital bills are totally unrealistic, charging astronomical prices because the hospital bean counters think they are sharper than the insurance company bean counters. I once saw a cafeteria worker on my unit counting salt and pepper paper packets in the juice room, why would a hospital pay someone to do that? Every item in medical stock is charged to the patient either by removing a sticker and placing it on the chart, or by pulling it from a big expensive machine using a secret code. Even medications are removed from a machine, and since most medicines are timed sometimes a line of nurses are standing in front of the machine waiting their turn. Just think what a confused patient can do to a nurse's work schedule. He shits the bed, go to the supply room at the end of the hall to sign out a diaper. Go to the linen supply cart to get linen, meanwhile, he has pulled off the monitor. Go to the medical supply room to get new monitor pads to reapply, it's medication time, he throws the meds onto the floor, and pours the water into the bed. Go to the pharmacy on another floor to get replacement meds. You have to show the meds that were thrown on the floor, so you have to find them wherever they went. And imagine you have six of these patients all doing the same thing. After your shift you sit in the parking lot for 30 minutes until the pain dies down enough for you to drive the car.

Doctors come to the floor for ten minutes and write an order, and it says to prepare the patient for heart surgery in the AM. The order reads shave the patient from chin to ankles, and have them sign a surgical permit specifying this and that, in medical terminology. Writing the order takes five minutes, shaving a patient can take a minimum of an hour or maybe two hours. Doctors cannot make money writing, they can make it by operating, so, the RN is ordered to help the doctor get the patient prepped so the doctor can get the big payback for his work on the OR table.

Some doctors make a career out of visiting other doctors long term patients in nursing homes. They have no staff, no office, no nurse, and no associates. Every dollar they make goes in their pocket. They use a computer, a fax machine hooked to their cell phone, and their car. They drive to the nursing home, see the patient, dictate the visit into their phone, send medication orders from their fax machine, print entries from their cell and fax, and off they go in a few minutes to the next patient, they make a killing.

They have figured how to beat the system using their brain and the best modern equipment, and the patient has any and all work done by the nurse. These doctors don't cheat, or try to get over on any patient, render good care, and don't need to bend rules to make their money. They take all comers, will travel within a reasonable area, and do what other doctors are loath to do, which is visit nursing home patients. I found working with them a pleasure because they were the model of efficiency with no bullshit attached, and they see multiple patients in the same building on the same day, or evening. Many of them prefer to work in the evening because traffic is less, family has gone home, patients are usually around their rooms, and they have all day off every day. As a matter of fact they were the only pleasant efficient thing I witnessed working in a nursing home.

The title almost says it all. On the floor where I worked in the hospital, we took a little survey to find the average age of our patients. The final number that we ended up with was 87. At 87 the bulk of the patients had some type of dementia, or total dementia, which posed a major problem for the nursing staff. Of course, the doctors spent as little time with the patients as they could, they did all their talking on their feet heading back out the door, but the nurses had to live with the patient for a 12 hour shift. Day shifts were bad but night shifts were the worst. Even the patients that were oriented during the day flipped a switch when the sun went down and became demented too. Of course, a nurse once receiving a group of patients, kept those patients every day until their time off, and sometimes two days later they would receive them back if they were still admitted to the hospital. Being a male nurse, of course, I would always have the rooms far down the hallway as far away from everything as they could get me, and any other male nurses working, because the female charge nurse always took care of the women.

Admitting a demented patient was always fun. It was really more fun if the family member was with them (usually) because I couldn't assess mental faculties of the patient because the family always answered the questions I asked before the patient had a chance to think and respond.

Sometimes I would ask the family member to hold up on their answers and allow the patient to respond. Almost always the patient would repeat the question back to me and smile and begin a silly laugh. They would do this to try and defer the response because their brain was gone and they couldn't answer the simplest direct question. They could tell a story about something that happened 50 years ago, but the direct question would throw them, they couldn't think. I knew then what I had on my hands for as long as they were on my unit/floor. Demented patients take many forms and some are really unpleasant.

First there are the rat, bug, it's looking at me group. These put on the call light or grab you when you are in the room and point out a spot near the ceiling and wall usually at a corner of the room. They whisper to you that there are (you name it, pick a bug, animal, person here) looking at them. They point at it and whisper so the (you name it) can't hear them, but you can. At first, I would try to prove that there was nothing there, but it was useless, they saw it and believed it. Usually after three days in the hospital the visions would vanish and the patient would become somewhat normal.

Second were the drinkers, they all had "just one or two very small drinks before supper." This group was a huge problem if they were still in the hospital on the third day after admission. On the third day they went into DT's (withdrawal from alcohol addiction) some hospitals let the patients have wine or beer with their meals which removed the threat of DT's. Others, like most of the hospitals, forbade any type of alcohol and the patients went nuts. Of course, the physician's, were very slow to prescribe a drug like Haldol to curb the symptoms. The patients would go through hell along with the nurses, doing every gyration that you could think of. Sweating, yelling, tearing, pulling, moaning, screaming, terror, and panic to name a few of the minor ones. Since I worked on a cardiac unit, every patient had a small heart monitor with wire leads connected to patches on their chest. Oh my GOD was this a fun thing, just try and find where the patient put the monitor after they pulled it off. Holy shit, sometimes they were ingenious in hiding the monitor in the most ridiculous spots. The patients would go for days sometimes forgetting that they were attached to the thing, and all of a sudden, they would "discover" it and pull it off. Monitors went everywhere in the hospital. They were hidden in a napkin on the food tray, thrown in the trash, thrown in the toilet, secreted in the bed under the covers, placed in the bedside table drawer, and anywhere else you can think of. We had a person called a monitor tech, watching the monitors for cardiac problems who would alert the nurse when the monitor signal disappeared, but you were not in a position to immediately run to the room to put them back on the monitor. Remember, these patients were not unstable patients, and this was not a CCU unit it was telemetry, and many patients that were on tele really did not need to be. The hospital tried to keep the tele beds occupied because they made more money than on a medical surgical floor.

Almost all the patients had hearing aids, false teeth, and eye glasses. I would answer a patients' call light and the patient would ask "what did I do with my (fill in the blank)" First you had better check the chart because all the possessions are listed there. If you were lucky there would be no listing for the item. If you were unlucky, you were in for another search mission because the patient would not remember where or what they did with it. I placed a call to the kitchen for a set of false teeth. Patients would place them on the food tray wrapped in a napkin and away they went. The kitchen said that they had some teeth and would send them up. When I received them, I gave them to a woman patient who quickly put them in her mouth. They happened to be men's teeth and she looked hilarious with this gigantic smile. I wish I had a picture of her it was really funny.

Sometimes, patients can catch the nurse off guard, and the nurse can be attacked and disabled for life if they are not really alert. Three incidents come to mind immediately, one when I was in college. We were having a work experience caring for nursing home patients. Two female students were given the task of showering a male patient. This task called for the patient to be placed in a rolling PVC chair and rolled into the shower after it was adjusted for temperature. What the students didn't know was that the patient had Hydrophobia. (a fear of water) An ailment common in the elderly because of a fear of slipping and falling on a wet surface. I was working across the hall from the shower room when I first heard a loud commotion. The commotion was disturbing because there was loud shouting, and some screaming, so I thought I had better investigate. When I opened the door and looked into the shower stall, I saw both the nurses on the floor of the shower with a quite large man standing over them kicking and stomping on them as hard as he could. He obviously had the upper hand, and both nursing students were on their backs using their hands and feet in an attempt to block the blows.

I immediately charged the old man, body blocking him away from the students and forcing him into the shower chair, and we both crashed into the back shower wall. He was off balance and was almost sideways into the shower chair where I knew he was vulnerable. I quickly got behind the chair and forced him to remain seated through his struggle, I knew I had him, and he couldn't do anything while seated. The two students got to their feet and started pushing him out of the shower room, the shower was over, and everyone was wet in the process.

The next incident was one of my friends working next to me was tasked with starting an IV on a difficult and sometimes violent patient. Usually two or three and sometimes even more nurses are needed to restrain the patient while we proceed to accomplish the orders for a patient. I asked Vince if he needed help but he said that he would be OK. He proceeded into the room with the IV kit but the female patient was ready for him. He set the kit down on the bed while he explained to the patient that he needed to place an IV in her arm because the doctor had ordered an IV medication. He bent over to put a tourniquet on her arm and she hauled off with a roundhouse punch aimed directly at his jaw. She missed slightly and clipped him on the side of the face, because he had seen it coming at the last minute and tried to move away. He was stunned by the blow but he recovered and grabbed her wrist as the next blow was already on its way. He wound up holding both hands and calling for a set of restraints which we had at the ready. With help he restrained the patient from delivering further blows and started the IV.

The third attack was around the corner of the hall in the last room before the doors to CCU. I was in an adjoining hallway but I heard the male nurse crash to the floor of the room. I went to the door of the room and saw a patient on his feet at the foot of the bed, and the nurse unconscious face down on the floor bleeding profusely from a head wound. The patient was sporting a nice wooden cane held by the rubber end using the bent handle as a striking instrument. He was very close to both the nurse and me, and was fully ready to strike the next blow. Keeping a keen eye on the patient, I reached down and grabbed an outstretched arm of the nurse and drug him out of the room, and out of immediate danger. I pushed the door open to the CCU and yelled for help for the nurse. As staff rushed to help him, I resolved to go after the patient and restore order. Still poised to strike I figured that I could get to him before he could complete the circular swing he had planned. I also knew that if I got inside of the arc he could not get the hit he wanted. I immediately charged him and made contact before he could complete the swing as I had figured. Once I made contact, even though we were both the same size I knew I could have my way with him because the elderly have balance issues. I knew that once I knocked him off balance his fear of falling would take over and he would forget abought the fight, and I was right. His fight was over, and in a couple minutes I had more help than I needed. The nurse who suffered the blow to the head from the cane never recovered. He was admitted to the hospital and developed neurological issues from the blow that never resolved, ending his career.

There used to be a way to handle patients that were so demented that they could not be controlled without dosing them with medications that would dope them up. One other way was essential tie them to the bed with restraints until they sort of "got the idea." Those days gradually were phased out, and a sort of patients bill of rights became the norm. Of course, chemically restraining the patients is a lot more sophisticated now, leading to better compliance. I have seen the elderly pull against restraints continuously for several days both night and day. A normal person would experience fatigue after an hour or so, but these patients can go on for days without wearing down. After three days they collapse and fall asleep sometimes sleeping for 48 hours after one of these events. When they fall asleep, we would remove the restraints so they could have complete freedom of movement. When they would awaken, they almost never needed the restraints reapplied.

Pulling out tubes is always a problem for elderly people with various stages of dementia. Many times, after a patient had wet the bed repeatedly the nurse would ask for a Foley catheter to be inserted to preserve the skin from being ruined by urine. In men and women, we would insert a Foley catheter which emptied into a bag which was hooked to the lower bed rail. The Foley stayed in position by inflating a balloon with 10 cc of saline lodged in the bladder. When the patient got out of bed to walk someone would have to unhook the bag and carry it along. At night the patient would turn on the call light and the nurse would assist them to the bathroom. It got very labor intensive when the patient got out of bed unassisted in the dark and walked to the bathroom. Checking on the patient especially men, the nurse would find the catheter stretched out on the floor leading to the bathroom with the fluid filled ball resting at the end of it. From that point there would be a trail of blood droplets leading to wherever the patient had gone. In effect, the patient had reamed out his prostate himself by pulling the inflated ball through his penis. Often you would think that someone was murdered in the room the blood trail was so extensive. Reinsertion of the catheter usually stemmed the flow enough to clot the bleeding off.

Nasogastric tubes are meant to relieve the pressure on the stomach and small intestine caused by a stopped up digestive track. When the intestines stop functioning, the fluids build up in the system until they reach the stomach, once they reach the stomach and fill it up, the patient gets very sick. If you insert a tube into the stomach and connect it to suction the patient feels better very quickly. When a patient is alert and oriented you can explain why the tube is placed, and they leave it alone. The tube is in the esophagus and does not interfere with breathing at all, the breathing tube is the trachea. Placing an NG (nasogastric)tube can be a difficult experience in a patient with dementia, they have no idea what's going on, and they will yank out the tube as soon as you turn around. I placed several tubes in a patient, and had him pull them out as soon as I left the room. It was becoming a time consuming experience that I was tiring of quickly. As a last resort I went to supply and retrieved 10 NG tubes and placed the packs at the bedside. I told the patient that he could pull the tubes out as much as he wanted and I would keep putting them back in, and we would see who got tired of it first. He looked at the pile of tubes on the table and looked back at me but said not a word. I left the room and he never pulled another tube out during his admission.

Bed climbers are a real problem in any hospital environment. They go over the rails usually at night, take off everything and want to wander around, usually showing up at the nurses station naked. One night I had several and they were really annoying to the point of almost being funny with their exploits. I found one of my patients naked walking down the hallway toward me, and redirected him back to his room. I put his gown back on him and placed him back into bed with the covers pulled up to his neck. I put out his light that I was using to dress him again, and said goodnight. I left the bedside and walked to the door and before I exited out the door, I turned to get a last look at the patient. When I turned, I bumped into something that was so close behind me it startled me. It was the same patient I had just put into bed a few moments before, he had gotten over the rails and followed me to the door without me hearing a sound. Once the full picture came to me about what had happened, I had to laugh.

Shitters are something that no nurse wants for a patient. Some shit all over the bed but say nothing. You smell shit in the room so you pull back the covers and there it is a brown stinking mess for you to clean up with the patient sitting square in the middle of it. One of my patients was wearing underwear and a T shirt brought from home when he messed the bed. The real problem arose when I tried to get the T shirt off without pulling the crap up his back and over his head, and he had a full head of hair. Very daintily I gathered the shirt up and started to maneuver it up toward his head. The shirt was so loaded that like all best plans this one was a complete failure and the shit got all over him. All the while he kept asking me if I could get him his job back at General Motors. That was an hour of hard labor in the worst conditions which set my med pass back an hour making me run around to try and make up for lost time. Can you imagine what happens to a nurse who has four shitters out of their 6 patients?

Helping patients to the bathroom is fraught with risk. You have to be behind the patient holding their gown shut and while drawing it tight you lend them a lot of support to walk. We also had a gait belt to hold which was around their waist, remember, patients don't have handles on their bodies. You have to walk close to the patient to maintain control over their motion. Being close leaves your lead foot at risk. At risk for what you say, shit dropping on your foot and sock. I used to wear white clogs which could be thrown in the washing machine. The socks were routinely discarded, and I bought the clogs three pair at a time for obvious reasons. More than once I took my pants home in a wet plastic bag and got scrub pants from the operating room to wear for the rest of the day. Taking care of shitters is problematic to say the least.

You walk into the room and the patient is on the floor, you have no idea how they got there, everything in the room looks normal. Remember, you can't get them up without loads of help. If the patient could get up themselves, they would have done that already. Once you assure yourself that they are not injured, you need lots of help because there is nothing to get hold of on a person to lift them, it's like they are made up of blubber and spaghetti. What you need is a bath blanket and four people. The patient is rolled onto their side, and the bath blanket is tucked under them. You then roll the patient back to the other side and pull the bath blanket out from under them which puts them in the center of the blanket. The four helpers roll up the blanket to make a hand hold and you all lift at once. Getting four able bodied nurses capable of lifting 50 lbs. or more is a feat in itself. Who do you think falls on the floor? Is it the 95 lb. old lady, or the 300 lb. old man, I'll let you guess.

NOT AS EASY AS YOU THINK

When I say fight him into the chair, I mean fight him into the chair

Many patients with dementia are kept at home until a situation develops that causes them to be moved elsewhere. In this case it was a 70's year old large male who was being taken care of by his loving wife. Lately, he had become belligerent and she was becoming more and more afraid that he would attack her and cause serious injury. He had already attacked her, and caused minor injuries like bruises, sore hands and fingers, and others. She discussed this with her husband's physician and he decided to admit the husband to the hospital while he looked for a place to put the husband. Naturally, being a patient that wanted to fight over everything, he was assigned to me to see to his care.

The patient did not like the change in surroundings, and made it well known that he was not going to comply with anything asked of him. While in the hospital a patient needs to be compliant with care, that means that he cannot disrupt the care of other patients, which this man was prone to doing. He was very obnoxious and loud, and other patients wanted to know who the hell is making all that ruckus. Eventually, in the absence of chemical restraints (medication that puts him to sleep) we had to place him into a vest which secured him to the bed to keep him from trying to get up and falling to the floor. He resolved that if we did not take off the vest, he would mess the bed which would force us to take off the vest to get him up. (remember, this man was a brute, and physical danger was always present when you were anywhere close to him) Sure enough true to his promise he messed the bed deliberately, and I had to get him up and place him in a chair to change the bed. I got together two other male nurses and we were able to fight him into the chair and affixing the vest ties to the frame of the chair to hold him in the chair. (when I say fight him into the chair, I mean fight him into the chair, male nursing isn't for sissies) None of us were injured in the process, although GOD knows he tried. He was so pissed that he issued various threats which included ripping my arms and legs off when he got out of the vest. (remember, this patient was not physically sick, he was mentally ill) The hospital was for patients with a variety of illnesses, but harboring violent patients capable of inflecting serious injury and even death on the staff is stretching the health care dollar a little much.

Once placed in the chair, watching me change the bed infuriated this guy to the point of yelling at the top of his lungs, HELLLLP, HELLLLP, HELLLP over and over again. (remember, I still had to clean him up, which would take a minimum of four or five male nurses to do) Each time he yelled HELLLLP it was louder than the time before, and I worked on the bed as fast as I could to be able to get him back into the bed again and stop his yelling out. After about the 30th time yelling at the top of his lungs, he fell silent in the middle of a yell, uttering HELugh, and was quiet. I was astonished, he coded right there in the chair, and went silent as his heart stopped dead, and I mean dead.

I mashed the code button, and set about untying the vest straps from the chair frame as I waited to get help to get him out of the chair to perform CPR on him. In a minute help flooded into the room, and we were able to get him muscled into the bed and begun the code. All the efforts were for naught he was irrevocably dead. This was one time that I was glad to see the struggle end. Nursing is tough enough with all the manual labor involved, but fighting with patients goes well beyond the scope of employment. I saw officers in the jail handle violent inmates, and they have special armored clothing, helmets, face protection, gloves, shields, and sprays. The nurses have only their bare hands, and are forced by physicians and administration to handle patients that are every bit as violent as those inmates in the jail. Demented crazy patients are just as big and powerful as any inmate in the jail and just as vicious. You haven't lived until you have had an old lady with yellow long jagged fingernails caked with every kind of nasty shit under them scratch the hell out of you while you try to clean her up after she just crapped into the bed. Old ladies love long pointed dirty fingernails and toenails, and they know how to use them against nurses, plus they bite too.

BLUE BLANKET (DON'T READ THIS ALONE)
The blanket was brought to the home by a family

Mental health issues abound in the United States, and have grown worse since the Mental Health Act of 1980. That act closed most of the mental institutions in the country and placed mental health patients into community based group homes, or specialized hospital wings, or units. The act also gave the mentally ill a "bill of rights" which allowed them to refuse treatment and prescribed medications. Now you know why there are so many mentally ill people standing on street corners with cardboard signs. Eventually, the mentally ill find their way into either jail or a hospital, and that just speaks to the younger population living on the streets. The older mentally ill population usually ends up in a rehab center. (these used to be called nursing homes, until the elderly realized that they were committed for life. The nursing home sign was removed, and a rehabilitation center sign was erected and the refusals vanished because the elderly were stuck on the nursing home name, and didn't realize that it was the same place).

I took a job supervising two wings in a rehab center for six months, I couldn't take much more. There were volumes of problems with supervising employees working under the duress that environment provides. All of the people in my two wings were put there by their families, and it was easy to understand why. The families couldn't deal with them 24 hours a day, and paid us to do it. The staff, both LPN's and nurses looked for any excuse, or any lie to stay home from working their shift. The pay was not bad, but there was no incentive to work in an environment where every single patient either shit their pants, or shit in the bed. That meant clean up in aisle 7 took place all day and most of the night.

The ones that could talk, always knew to tell us "I made a mess again" when they had finished shitting.

I had a group sitting directly in front of the nurses station continuously asking for the time, every two minutes for hours on end. Try to chart on a patient with 6 people calling out "excuse me, excuse me, excuse me, excuse me", for the entire shift. They wanted to know the time because they were all waiting for their parents to come and get them to take them home. There was no use talking rationally to the patients, they were right back asking the same question as soon as you finished talking. I started pushing their wheelchairs all the way to the end of the other wing, which gave me about 15 minutes to get some of my work done, before they were able to scoot back and start all over again with "excuse me."

Once every month I had to examine every patient on the two wings, which included blood pressure pulse, temp, physical eval, and check their skin for problems. (skin issues will get the business sued, so keeping the skin clean and nice and pink was essential." The semi-comatose patients were the worst to try and assess, because as soon as they were touched, they assumed that they were being assaulted and fought like hell. I tried everything to get a B/P on them, sometimes taking almost ½ hour in some cases with the patient fighting me all the way. I tried on the leg, and that was worse because they kicked all the time. Pulses were better because most of the time I could watch their neck and see it throbbing. Whatever you did it was time consuming and fraught with peril for the RN. You could never be sure how the patient would strike, so you had to be alert, and able to move quickly before the knee, heel, or elbow crashed into your face as you leaned in to hear the beats through your stethoscope. Many times, I was able to block the blow, but if you do it long enough, they eventually get you.

Feeding time is a totally different experience, where all of the residents that can feed themselves go to the dining room, or are wheeled to the dining room to eat. The food is served on trays, and I used to help the few aids serve the trays to the residents. It was maddening every day, because there were residents that said "this is not what I ordered" or "take it away I'm not hungry" or "my mother is bringing me something special." You could spend an hour with each one trying to convince them that it was their food tray, all to no avail, they were adamant in their confusion.

Then there was the woman who had a pureed diet ordered by the physician and refused to eat the pureed food. Her relatives were able to get some doctor to let her have a non-pureed diet, and she choked on every other bite of food. When I say choked, I mean purple face, inability to inhale, the works. There was nothing to be done, she had an order to let her choke until she was able to clear the airway herself. The residents would hear her choke every meal, and would yell at me "you're a nurse, do something." Once she had possession of the food, there was no way to get it back, except possibly the Heimlich maneuver which entailed throwing her onto the floor. She always cleared her throat, and went on to take the next bite, and start all over again. Then the residents would look at me and again say "you're a nurse, do something." And the resident who refused her tray would pipe up with; "this is the worst restaurant I've ever been to, where is the meal I ordered." And the woman at the next table would yell "shut up with this noise, I'm trying to eat", and another "where's my mother with my food." A few families would come every day to feed their relative, and that would be a treat watching them taste everything on the tray before they spooned it into the relative's mouth. If the relative was finally full, the person feeding them would spin the tray around and finish off the food themselves. Nothing went to waste when the relatives were present at mealtime. One day everyone was excited because stuffed peppers were on the menu. When supper came everyone was licking their chops until the trays came out of the kitchen. The cook took raw peppers and stuffed them with the cooked meat, you should have seen the faces when they spotted the raw peppers, it was priceless. That day the cook took the brunt of abuse from the patients, and they left the other staff alone.

Then there were the relatives who liked to call on the phone to "check on Mrs. XXX." They would ask to speak to "my mothers nurse." I would answer the phone, and when they asked to speak to the mothers nurse, I would tell them that the nurse was busy passing medications. (and they were) The caller would say that they wanted to speak to the nurse anyway, and I would again say that the nurse is busy. Well, one black woman who called every day after work got really pissed at me and came to the Center to tell me off. She wanted to argue at the nurses station, but I asked her to step onto the porch and brought a nurses aide with me. (I brought a second person to verify the conversation should it come to that) The relative told me that she would go to the administrator over the issue of her wanting to talk to her mother's nurse. I told her that medication mistakes are made when the nurse passing medications keeps getting interrupted. I informed her that she could come to the center any time she wanted and could talk to the nurse as she rendered care according to her duties. However, she would not be able to drag the nurse away from the care of patients to answer mundane questions. The woman stormed off in a huff heading straight for the administrator's office. When she was through with the administrator she returned to the wing and puttered around with her mother in the day room all the time glaring at me with side looks, then she left. I found out that her trip to the administrator was not what she expected. He listened to her argument, and asked her if she was unsatisfied with the care her mother was receiving. He then told her that if she was unsatisfied, she could pull her car up to the front door of the building, and he would personally load her mother into the car. He said she could then take her mother wherever she thought she could get better care than she was receiving here. He further informed her that he could get a hundred patients before he could find one good nurse to care for them. I guess that shut her up, especially when he showed her the waiting list he had for her mother's room. She didn't call anymore, and she didn't try to bully the staff again either.

A daughter of one of the patients had successfully pulled off a scam on the government, and the nursing home. They had bilked everyone, and hid the mother's assets from everyone. The mother owned a large home, and a piece of property near the beach, I believe it was a motel. Her daughter and husband both worked, and lived in a condo, with no children. When the mother showed signs of dementia, the daughter investigated what was necessary to get the mother into a full care nursing home. At the time, you had to present tax returns for about three years prior to admittance for review. The home would review the persons assets, and decide on a price. The daughter, armed with this info began to transfer all the mother's assets into her own name. She moved into the mother's big home and transferred the small condo into her mother's name. She did the same with everything the mother owned after declaring the mother incompetent to handle her own affairs. She looked after the mother for the required time, and when she was sure that she was in the clear she applied for the nursing home care. The mother's assets were a small condo, and a thin bank account, which the nursing home based their charges on plus her social security payment. Meanwhile the daughter quit her job and her husband quit his job because the motel was sold for the neighborhood of four million. Little did the husband know what was in store for him down the road.

The mother was admitted to the nursing home, and the daughter came every day with her husband dragged along, to sit with the mother and fuss over her. The daughter had a daily routine of activities for the mother which depended on her husband doing the grunt work like lifting, carrying, holding, dragging, and manhandling the mother. All the time the mother had no idea who the daughter was. In between tasks the husband liked to talk to me, and would usually get a chair and sit with me in the dining room off to the side, while his wife tried to feed the mother. He wanted to live vicariously through me, asking me what I had to eat last night, where I bought it, how did I prepare it, where was I going on vacation etc. He virtually drooled on himself when I described some fish filets I had cooked last evening. His daily routing was always the same, visiting the nursing home daily, and returning home alone to make supper which was only a cold salad every day. After he made the salad he would return to the nursing home and retrieve his wife, who had tucked the mother in for the night. The next day he would start again, and again having a cold salad every night.

One day he asked me if I thought his wife was going to have the same problems as his mother-in-law because she was the spitting image of the mother. I told him the truth as I saw it, the daughter was developing subtle signs associated with the mother's disease process. He then asked me what he could do to help the wife. I told him that the routine his wife developed, a routine of "social isolation" would do her in even faster. He was concerned but nothing was going to change, and he knew it, so he just plodded on following his wife around the nursing home following orders. The wife had appropriated millions and it did neither of them any good whatsoever, they spent all their days in the nursing home, and went home to cold salads.

The next happening borders on the macabre, it is the story of the blue blanket. Long before I came to work in the nursing home a story circulated among the nurse's aides. The story centered around the mysterious blanket kept by one of the aides in her locker. The blanket was a harbinger of special life or death properties. All of the aides were afraid of the blanket, and afraid to touch it on pain of death.

The story goes like this; the blanket was brought to the home by a family to cover their family member who was dying, with only days to live. They wanted the patient to have something from home to comfort him in his last hours. The aide placed the blanket onto the patient even though he was covered with supplied linen. The blanket was unfurled over all on the bed, and was applied every night and removed from the room during the day. Every night the blanket was tossed to the floor by the unconscious patient, how it happened no one knows, it was told that the patient was totally unable to toss the blanket off, and all the other linen stayed in place undisturbed. This went on for four nights, and on the fifth night the blanket stayed on, and the patient died. The family refused the blanket after the death and it was secured by the aide who had cared for the patient. Patient after patient I was told had done the same thing and finally died with the blanket on. After each death, the aide would carefully fold the blanket and place it in her locker to await the next use.

We received a hospice patient who only had days to live, and the aides talked "is he ready for the blue blanket" the aide with the blanket said she would bring it out the next night. I was working when the aide came through the wing with the folded blanket, trailing every aide in the place like a funeral cortege. I don't believe in all that mystical shit, but I tagged along to see the ceremony. The aide unfurled the blanket and floated it over the patient in bed. The ceremony was over, and we all went about our tasks, I got a kick out of the group all afraid of the blanket, but I didn't touch it either. Later, before the end of my shift, I went to check on the patient and the blanket. The Goddam blanket was on the floor, and the covers were totally undisturbed, and the patient was totally comatose. How the hell that blanket got on the floor I had no clue, and no one entered the room but me, they were all afraid to go in there. I called the aide, and she retrieved the blanket saying that he was not ready. I was off the next night, but it was noted that the blanket was on the floor again. The next night, the blanket stayed on all night and the patient was dead before daylight broke. I often wondered if the blanket is still on that wing of the nursing home doing its job.

WATCH OUT HERE IT COMES
He had begun back-talking the grandmother

When I did home health for a hospital based home health care agency I received all of the cases in a ghetto area not far from the offices. Since I was a male nurse, the women running the agency used me to go where the female nurses refused to go. It was all money to me so as long as I was making dollars I really didn't care, plus some of the cases were easier to do. The only concerns I had were, would the car get stolen while I was in the home, or would the car get broken into.

In this case I was sent to do a routine blood pressure check on an elderly black lady who suffered from very high blood pressure. She had just been discharged from the hospital after a week, getting her blood pressure stabilized on several new medications. She greeted me at the door, and let me inside because she had been informed that I would be along to keep a check on her. She was somewhat excited to see a nice "white boy" coming to visit her, which had never happened before. She wanted to talk, so while I did my tasks, she rambled on about her life. She told me that she was a widow, and her husband had died over twenty years earlier. She said that she had one child a son, who married, and produced two little boys, which she loved very much. Further, she said that she was having all sorts of problems trying to raise the two boys herself, because her son and his wife were both put in prison for dealing drugs. She said that they had been in jail over ten years, and the oldest boy was all grown up. Both of the boys lived with the grandmother because she owned a house where they could live, and they would be able to attend school every day from home. She kept on, telling me that she had been having some trouble with the older boy who was attending middle school. He was hanging out with boys who were influencing him in a bad way, and he had begun back-talking the grandmother. Up to this point she was able to control him, but now he was taller than her, and was hovering over her and trying to intimidate her. He was probably part of the cause of her recent blood pressure problems.

Just before her admission, things with the grandson had come to a head. She was in the kitchen preparing supper, when the oldest boy told her he was going out. Knowing that he had not done his homework, the grandmother told him to stay home until supper. He balked at that request, and decided that he would do as he pleased, and he was not staying home.

The grandmother informed him that he would do as she said, because he lived in her home, and she was the boss here. He approached her in the kitchen, and the conversation turned into an ugly confrontation at this point. The grandson retorted with the statement "I ain't taking no orders from no old lady." This infuriated the grandmother, who told him "you think because your bigger than me that I can't kick your ass"? The grandson said "I'd like to see you try" and turned on his heel walking away toward the front door. At that point the grandmother picked up a black iron frying pan and hurled it at the grandson, striking him on the back of his head. He was unconscious before he hit the floor. The other grandson jumped up from the kitchen table where he was doing his homework to check on his brother. He yelled "grandma, you killed him dead."

That did not phase the old lady, who said, "let that be a lesson to both of you, you talk to me with respect, or you'll get the same thing."

The older grandson eventually awakened, with a big knot on his head, and realized that he had been clobbered by the grandmother. She told him that if he ever talked to her again like that, she would wait until he went to bed and she would bring that frying pan down hard on his face. I don't think he ever got out of line again, and her blood pressure was fine.

THE HONEYMOONER

He would have to take the wound vac with him

When working as a home health care coordinator, I received a referral to setup a patient in his late 50s. The patient had an abscess on his leg that was infected with MRSA. The doctor wanted the patient to have a wound vac and six weeks of IV antibiotics. I looked at the patient chart, and he had excellent insurance. I thought this would be a routine referral until I spoke to the patient. He was agreeable to home care, but he wanted to set it up in North Carolina. I have setup home care for people out of state before but these patients were visitors or seasonal residents. They were established with a primary care physician in their home state. What I would do was (with their permission) call their doctor in their home state and inform him that his patient was going to need home care. Next, I would fax the chart to their out of state doctor's office. The following day I would call the physician's office and ask what agency they would like to use? Then I would call and fax the chart to the home care agency the out of state doctor wanted to use.

I asked the patient if he had a doctor in North Carolina. The patient said he did not. My next question why do you want to go to North Carolina? He told me he had been corresponding with a prisoner in a New York state prison. They decided to get married upon her release from prison. She was scheduled to be released on Saturday (the day I first spoke to the patient was Tuesday) and she was to fly into Atlanta. He would meet her at the airport. After that they would drive to North Carolina and get married, and honeymoon in North Carolina. He planned a month long honeymoon in a cabin in the Great Smokey Mountains. He had already placed a deposit on the cabin rental. I told him

I could not help him unless he had a physician who had a license to practice medicine in North Carolina. I told him no home care agency in North Carolina would accept him as a patient unless he had a doctor who was license to practice medicine in the state, I then left the room.

The following day he told me his brother who lives in North Carolina got him a doctor and a home health care agency. I first called the doctor's office. I was told the doctor might accept him as a patient, but only after he examined him. After speaking to the doctor's office nurse, I called the home care agency. They said they will be willing to accept him if his insurance checks out and if he can get a physician in North Carolina.

I returned to the patient's room and told him you have no firm commitment from the doctor in North Carolina. After he examines you, he may or may not accept you as a patient. You do not even have an appointment for an examination. Assuming you can get in to see him on Monday, and he accepts you as a patient, the earliest you will receive home care is on Tuesday. This means if you discharge on Friday, you will miss three doses of your antibiotics. Your wound vac dressing needs to be changed three times a week. You will also miss your Monday dressing change.

I asked him if he thought of the logistics of what he was trying to do. I told him the wound vac had a battery that lasted four hours. I told him it is an eight hour drive to Atlanta. The wound vac could be plugged into your cigarette lighter in the car, but what happens if the car breaks down. I told him any stops along the way; to use the restroom, pump gas or get something to eat, he would have to take the wound vac with him. Think about carrying the wound vac around the Atlanta airport while you are waiting for your girlfriend's plane to land. I asked him, "do you think you are going to have a romantic honeymoon hooked to a wound vac "?

He asked me "what should I do." I told him he should remain at his house until his treatment was finished. He should get in contact with his girlfriend and tell her about his illness. Tell her the honeymoon is off until your treatment is finished. Instead of going to Atlanta she should come to

Florida. Next, he should call the people who he gave the deposit for the cabin and explain his situation and see if he can get his deposit back.

In this story we have a perfect example of a patient's family member hearing only what he wanted to hear and not what was being said. The patient's brother did hear the doctor say I might accept your brother as a patient after an examination. His brother did not hear the representative of the home care agency tell him, we can accept your brother if he can get a doctor and if we are able to accept his insurance. What he did hear was the doctor and home care agency would accept his brother.

Eventually, he listened to reason and stayed at his home until his treatment was completed, his new bride made her way to join him there.

This story is also an example of a patient who does not think. He never thought about the difficulties in going to Atlanta and then to North Carolina. He did not consider the effects of his MRSA infection on his honeymoon.

MIRACLES DO HAPPEN
She was going on a trip with guess who?

I was working home health, seeing patients in their homes. One of my patients was the wife of a very caring man. The wife spent most of her day in either bed, or an easy chair, and appeared to be virtually an invalid. The husband did everything for his wife including, cooking, cleaning, shopping etc. When I visited her, she seemed very stable to me but always complained about chronic severe pain. Her blood pressure was always fine, her glucose finger stick was normal, so I cut her visits down to twice a week from every day. When I visited, I always had a few minutes to talk to the husband, who when cooking, always had on a woman's frilly apron. We used to joke about it, and sometimes I thought he wore it just so we could laugh about it.

He told me that this was his second marriage, and they had been married for 3 years. He said that his wife took ill with the chronic debilitating pain just after their marriage, and through the years had never seemed to get better, she just stayed the same. Home health was ordered because as he aged, he was falling further and further behind in his chores, shopping, etc, and he needed help with caring for his invalid wife. A home health aide was provided, who helped the wife with her bathing needs, and other patient related chores. She also had physical therapy to ambulate her on a walker in an attempt to keep her mobile.

This turned out to be a long term case and had been seen long before I came on the scene, I just picked up the case after the assigned RN stopped working for the agency. I had been on the case for several months, usually stopping to see them in the late morning just before lunch. I arrived as usual, and a different person (a neighbor) answered the door. I was surprised not to see the husband, and inquired of the neighbor where he was. I was surprised to learn that he had been found dead in bed that morning. The husband and wife occupied different bedrooms in the home. I went to see the wife, and she was in her normal position in a recliner, but not as upset as I thought she would be. I went through my usual tasks, and expressed my regret about the passing of her husband. When I left the home, I called the office to report the death of the husband to the case manager, and went on to the next patient visit. On the next visit day, I checked to make sure that we were still on the case, and was assured that nothing had changed. When I got to the home, a gentleman answered the door and let me in. I went through my usual tasks and found everything normal, as usual. The gentleman was described as a friend of the family who was available to help. As the next few weeks passed, the widow seemed to get much better, allowing me to cancel the home health aide. Eventually she was walking in the home, fully dressed, and really enjoyed having the gentleman friend around. After a couple of months, I was removed from the home entirely because the services were terminated on the widow's request, she was going on a trip with guess who.

YOU CAN THINK, THEY CAN'T THINK!

Everyone involved in the accident was killed but her

I reported to the nursing office for my assignment, and I was sent to a lockdown unit for brain damaged patients. These units are meant to contain patients that may be mobile, but do not have cognitive thought. (they can't think like you and me) They are prone to wandering, and locking down the unit assures everyone that they stay within prescribed boundaries. Brain damaged patients fall within certain groups, the largest of which are motorcycle riders. Almost half of the patients were drunk driving motorcycles at night, and had one vehicle accidents. (only the motorcycle was involved) They usually were going fast and misjudged a curve and ran off the road and crashed. Very few were wearing helmets, and those that were received closed head brain injuries. All of them in the unit had received severe brain injuries, and were alive in body only.

In one particular case a young man about thirty had a very pleasant wife, and a new baby, who came to spend time with him almost every day. The nurses on the unit explained that the wife had been beaten by the husband in drunken rages while she was pregnant. The husband was described as a "bad actor." This guy required complete care which was feeding, washing, changing, everything you could think of. His discharge was looming, and the doctor wanted to make arrangements for his placement in a facility. (there are human warehouses where patients are placed permanently until death) The wife objected, and wanted the patient sent home with her and the baby. She said she would provide all the care necessary for his well-being. Therefore, she was trained by the nurses in preparation for discharge. The feeling was that she was going to get even with the bastard for all the beatings she got from him. I'm willing to bet that what the nurses thought was the truth.

The second type of patients in the unit, were falls, where the patient struck their head really hard. This type of patient usually had a physical disability from the fall, and a closed head brain injury too. Unbelievably, most of these injuries were the do-it-yourself husbands, who always said "I'll just throw a ladder up, and do it myself it will only take a minute." There were more of this type than one would realize, I certainly didn't. They were usually not as bad as the motorcycle group, and could be led around like they were in a daze, and some would even follow simple instruction like "sit down."

The third type were a mix of automobile accident, bar fights, roofers, and bicycle rider-car collisions, but they were by far in the minority. One of the most notable cases in this group was a young woman in her twenties who was in a terrible car accident in Nevada. Both her and a friend were travelling at night on one of those highways with no speed limit when the accident occurred. Everyone involved in the accident was killed at the scene but her, and she was mangled in the wreckage and had to be extricated. From the looks of her, you would think she was at fault, because she at twenty something, was covered with grotesque tattoos. After seeing her, two things came to mind, a motorcycle gang, or a rock star groupie.

Nurses like to play sick jokes on each other when possible, so me being agency I was not familiar with this female patient. The staff nurses knew that this female had no inhibitions and would immediately offer me all kinds of sexual favors through her slurred speech. They were watching and waiting for me to get into the room to pass my meds and see if she needed any care that I would provide. As I made my rounds, they were watching me like a hawk when I entered her room. I approached the bed and the patient asked me if I had come to "get some." Me being a dumb ass, asked her "get some of what"? She flung back her covers revealing that she had pulled her gown up and was showing me her vagina. I heard a lot of giggling at that point and realized that I had been set up by the female nurses watching from around the doorway. They all knew what was going to happen with that patient. The worst part of the whole thing was I had a tough time all night wrestling with her trying to keep her from grabbing me in the wrong places, she was a trip. I was glad when that night was over, and although I was assigned there numerous times, I never had her again.

This group of stories brings to mind the story of a roofer who avoided the brain injury route by some quick thinking and manual dexterity. The roofer was working three stories up, on a shingle roof. He told me that there were strips of wood nailed to the bottom of the roof to prevent falling off. If you slid down the slope of the roof, your feet would catch the strip and stop the slide before you went over the edge. He had finished a section, and was walking along the roof to a new spot when he stepped on a loose shingle laying on top of the ones nailed down. The shingle slid and he went with it, falling onto the roof. He began to slide down the roof feet first, when to his horror he saw that there was no strip of wood there to stop his slide. His mind raced for the several seconds his slide took. He was trying to picture what was below the roof at that section of the property. He remembered a concrete walkway directly below, a small section of grass lawn, and a retention pond after the grass. As he slid, he thought that if he could hit the ground at the retention pond, he might survive the fall. When he reached the edge of the roof feet first, he pushed off as hard as he could from the edge of the roof with both hands hoping it would propel him the distance to the pond. When he pushed off hard, it had the effect of turning him over so his feet faced the building, and his head out toward the pond, he thought that this was a good, though unexpected thing. With his back toward the ground and his face toward the sky, he made his descent. He tried to look down as he saw that he had already passed the concrete walkway, and was over the grass plot. As the fall continued, he thought "I might make the pond" as he crashed to the ground halfway into the pond and halfway onto the lawn and tall grass at the end of the pond. His head splashed into the 10 in. deep water and soft muck in the pond, and he immediately knew he would be OK. He suffered a back injury and leg injuries, but he recovered and avoided the brain injury unit altogether.

THE JAIL

The nurse made it out and the guard caught the inmate

People who get locked up in jail are not going to get medical care even if they need it badly. The jail is not a place that wants to provide any medical care for a variety of reason that seem sound to them. The biggest reason they defer care, is because any patient sent to a hospital has to have a deputy sheriff accompany the inmate, and that is very costly. The second reason is hospitals are not free, so the sheriff has to pay for the hospital stay. Lets go over a few stories relating to either care, or lack of care, or complete ignorance and stupidity associated with no care provided. We all have to realize that inmates are in jail because they need to be punished, and the sheriff is there to make sure of that.

I was hired by the jail to serve as an RN in the various buildings where inmates are housed. There are essentially five areas, maximum security, minimum security, teens, women, and women with aids. A nurse can be assigned in any of the five areas depending on how much you suck up to the boss, an old floor supervisor who used to work in a big hospital but was fired because all the floor nurses wanted her gone. She ruled over the worst conglomeration of old know nothing, clap trap, incompetent, shit balls, I ever met. When I started, I was assigned to work in maximum security which required you to pass through a series of electrically locked confined areas to get inside. Once inside you were free to access most areas of the jail. I was to follow this old nurse (and I use the term loosely) who was treating inmates in a clinic setting. A guard would bring each inmate to see the nurse, and would stay in the room while treatment was given. A large black man was brought in who had a huge bandage on his entire back. I read that a female had thrown hot lie on him during a domestic dispute. The old nurse sat him down on a stretcher and walked behind him. She reached up grabbed the large dressing and ripped it off in one quick downward motion. The inmate yelled at the top of his lungs, and jumped off the stretcher and went for the nurse. The nurse must have known what was going to happen because she took off running as best she could. So, there were the three of them, the nurse with the head start, the inmate, and the prison guard all heading for the door. The nurse made it out and the guard caught the inmate at the door and brought him back into the room. He sat back down complaining about his treatment to the guard, who agreed with him. I looked at his back and it was a mess of raw meat with blood streaming down from various spots where the bandage was adhered. I cleaned him up, stopped most of the bleeding, and rebandaged according to the doctor's orders. When the guard took the inmate away the nurse returned to the room. I asked her why she tore off the bandage so viciously, and she replied that she didn't like that particular patient. We got into a disagreement over that, and she let me know that she was going to report my insolent behavior to the director. I decided that she was not going to get away with that, so I wrote a letter to the director telling her my side of the issue. Little did I know at the time, she was in real good with the director, and threatened to write me up but didn't do it. From that time forward I was a marked man.

The director decided that she would exile me from the maximum security building, and move me to the minimum security building. I was working there one evening when I was sent for urgently, to attend to an inmate who had passed out walking to chow. (the chow hall was in a free standing building between the women and minimum security and served both of them with food). The inmate was conscious so I did a quick workup on him where he sat on the steps of the building. He was in his sixties and normal weight, but his pulse was inadequate to support any activity, about 45 beats a minute. It seemed obvious that he needed a pacemaker. I reported this to the guards, and he was taken back to his cell. The guards restricted him to the cell and had another inmate bring him his food. There was no attempt to do anything for him other than restrict his movement so his pulse would not cause him to faint again. I also handed out the medications for that unit and he received nothing, so it could not have been his meds causing the problem.

I also had the responsibility for checking blood sugar's and giving insulin. Every day before dinner I would check the blood sugar of the male inmates per orders, and it was always off the charts. I would give the maximum dose of insulin and recheck it several hours later and again give another dose of insulin. There is nothing normal about this type of diabetic care, so I decided to look into the problem by asking one of the inmates with the highest blood sugar's where he worked in the jail. He informed me that he worked in the kitchen. I knew that food service was tightly controlled by the guards because, many of the guards ate in the cafeteria and the food was prepared by the inmates. You can just imagine what the inmates would do to the food the guards were eating, had they been left to their own devices. I walked over to the kitchen and talked to the sergeant in control. I took my diabetic list with me and showed it to him, asking where these men worked in food service. He pointed to a side room stating "they're in there." I walked to the door of the room and it all became apparent what was going on. The assholes were making sheet cakes. The jail had assigned the diabetic inmates to the kitchen making sheet cakes, so guess what they were snacking on. I immediately went back and wrote a memo to the nursing supervisor asking her to see to the reassignment of the diabetic prisoners to the laundry. Three days later I was summoned to the major's office to explain my memo to him. I didn't get to say a word, he informed me that I was never to communicate in writing ever again about jail experiences. He cited what could happen if a lawyer or newspaper would get their hands on my memo. He stated that they would be watching me going forward and he would recommend firing me if I didn't wise up. The diabetics stayed in the kitchen making sheet cakes and they moved me to the women's barracks. No one wanted to work the women's barracks because they were thought of as ball breakers, so I was on the shit list and was being punished.

The women's unit was selected to be the road crew, which means they go outside the enclosure with a truck and pick up debris on the side of the road. The women wanted a job, any job in the jail, because they got one day off their sentence for every day they worked in the jail. Inmates served 364 days maximum in the jail, any more and they were sent by bus to a prison to serve their time. One of the girls on the work crew came to sick call every evening asking for pain pills. All that was available was Tylenol, so I gave her two every night. Eventually, I got tired of constantly handing out Tylenol and wanted to know why she was in line every single evening wanting the pills. She reported that she was in severe pain after working on the road crew every day bending over picking up stuff. She also told me she was in a bad automobile wreck years ago that kept her in constant pain. I decided to look into her story, so I went up to the jail archives and found her previous charts. I went through them extensively as she, like the other inmates had been in jail for most of their lives. She had indeed been in a car wreck, she had been a passenger in a stolen car which had been chased by the police. The driver refused to stop and attained speeds over 100 mph when he lost control of the car and crashed. She was the only survivor, having been thrown out of the car through a side window. She suffered a shattered pelvis, two broken legs, a broken arm, three crushed vertebrae, and internal injuries. After reading her chart I sent her to see the jail physician to get stronger medications that would last longer than Tylenol. I also asked him to recommend she be sent to the laundry to work because the job was easier on her body. I gave the doctor a full accounting of her injuries. What I got back was a standing order for Tylenol every night, (which she was getting from me already) and to continue on the road crew.

As an aside to these stories I must inform you what transpires in the jail between inmates. I have seen male inmates after a fight in their cell pods. Some inmates file their fingernails into points and use them as knives on other inmates faces. Kicking an inmate from behind when they are at the top of a flight of metal steps causes a lot of damage to an inmate. The girls are especially brutal using their Melmac cups as weapons. When they line up for meals someone behind you will crack you over the head with a cup when the guards are occupied elsewhere. They also kick each other behind the knees to make the victim fall down. The culprit is never directly behind the victim, usually two or three people back for cover.

An inmate came to sick call with a severely infected foot. He was working on the kitchen detail washing trays after the meal. He worked on a line of men wearing a plastic bag over his socks, with a rubber boot on. The inmates were spilling water all over the place, and lots of it went down into the boots onto the inmate's feet. Of course, half the inmates had athlete's feet in the jail. This inmate had the front of his right foot amputated after a car wreck years before, and was left with only a heel. The heel was cracked, sopping wet, and covered with a fungus probably athlete's foot. He was in severe pain and could hardly walk on it, limping and trying to get around without putting it down. I sent him to see the jail doctor, who immediately sent him to the local hospital because the limb could possibly be amputated below the knee if good care was not given immediately. Of course, the jail would be liable, and a lawyer could have a field day with this one.

The inmate spent 4 weeks in the hospital and returned to the jail with his foot completely healed. Try and guess where the jail assigned him to work after his protracted recovery? I know where he was sent, because one month after he returned, he came to sick call limping again.

During my punishment time assigned to the women's wing I seemed to get along with the women pretty well. They were the same as anyone else. Once they understood that the nurse was going to give them a fair shake, and not blow them off, they settled down and became less of a problem. I had several patients that came to sick call and just really wanted to talk to someone. One was a girl who had scars all over her arms from knife fights with her husband. In fact, she was in jail because she won the last fight when he received a serious wound in his shoulder, but she was only stabbed in the forearm. She was sent in to see me to check on how it was doing, it was turning into a nice fat scar to go with the others.

Another was a young girl that had a long history of mental illness. She was a "cutter" who had multiple scars all up and down both arms from hacking away at herself for years. She told me that she was in a gang and her boyfriend cut her arms every time she disobeyed him, I knew she was lying.

A girl in solitary, that had been there for almost a year because she was mentally ill and incompatible with the rest of the female jail population, was to be released that day and refused to leave her cell. She had been incarcerated so long in the system, that she regarded her jailers as her family. She refused to leave the cell, holding the door shut because she had no where to go on the outside. She cried and cried and begged to stay, my shift ended and she was still begging the guards to let her stay there.

I met another young girl named Alice who was about 21 and a habitual drug taker, and was arrested for theft. She took a job working for a Maid Service that travels to people's homes to clean their houses. She would use the job to case people's homes for a later break-in and theft of the items she had spotted while cleaning. Of course, she had a long record of theft and was caught almost every time. She had a tooth ache in a molar and came to me for Tylenol. I looked at the tooth and there was a giant cavity, so I sent her to the jail dentist. Of course, I didn't know that he didn't fill teeth he extracted them. He took this young girl in the chair and pulled out her molar. In the year I worked at the jail she had 2 more teeth pulled by him.

The next criminal was a deaf girl who was a thief in cahoots with two others locked up with her. The deaf girl took a job in a factory assembling things on an assembly line. She worked there about three months, and used her time there to case the place for a midnight burglary. On the night they were burglarizing the office of the business, they were caught carrying business machines out, putting them in the trunk of the car they were using. The business had a silent alarm on the door they were using, so the police were notified when they sprung the door to gain entry. Every time they were rearrested it was like attending a party in the jail, they were surrounded by their friends anxious to know what they were caught doing. The jail was a subculture of society, a cult of criminals that had no intention of ever "going straight."

There was an epidemic of vaginal diseases in the women's section of the jail. Over half of the women were using vaginal suppositories to combat it, but they kept engaging in finger based sex which continued to re-infect them. When walking down the corridor in the women's section with a guard, I saw three women on a top bunk sitting there while another worked on them with hand sex. These girls were lousy at controlling any of their urges, many of them were prostitutes. I found that black men would pay to have sex with a white woman, but they expected it for free with a black woman.

The temperature in various sections of the jail depended on the conduct of the inmates. If the inmates behaved themselves, the temperature was set at 75 degrees. If there was any problem in the pod of inmates, the temperature would be set on 55 degrees, and the inmates would be curled up in their bunks with their one blanket freezing. You could tell immediately which pods were trouble areas by looking in the observation window. The inmates were for the most part well behaved, because they knew what would happen if they even laid a hand on another inmate, or a guard.

There was an isolation room single cell near the guard's outpost. It was used for punishment of inmates who had gone before an all guard tribunal. The tribunal would hear the complaint, and decide the punishment. Everything was handled in house, no judge, jury, paperwork, nothing but the tribunal. The inmate would receive a sentence to be carried out in the isolation cell at the guard station. The cell was unique, originally built to house an inmate with a contagious disease, it had its own heat and a/c system and high intensity lights. The inmate would be stripped of his clothes, given a bare mattress, and a thin blanket and placed into the cell. The lights would be on full 24 hours a day, and the temp would be lowered until the cell was like a refrigerator. There were no windows at all, and food was passed through a hole in the door which was only opened to feed the inmate, the room had a toilet with no seat (stainless steel) and a sink where water could be regulated by the guards. There was no concept of night or day, it was always day as far as the inmate was concerned. The inmate would serve the full sentence in that room unless another inmate had done something worse than the one in the room. If that was the case, the guy in the room would get his clothes back and be put back in the population, and the next inmate would take his place. No matter how mentally ill the inmate was, he would never want to go back in that isolation cell again, he learned his lesson well, freezing in that room.

Inmates would usually try to reason with each other in a rational fashion. Some inmates thought they were so bad ass that they wouldn't listen to reason. One case was when a bad ass was taking the food tray from a little defenseless guy with thick glasses. Several inmates asked "why don't you leave him alone"? The bad ass refused and even punched the poor guy in the face, and attempted to do it again. Five inmates stepped in, and when they were through the bad ass wouldn't recognize himself in the mirror. When the guards asked the bad ass what happened, he said he fell out of bed and hit his face on the floor. He knew that he would be put in isolation and was afraid of that.

We come to my last experience at the jail, the experience that sent me back outside working in real medicine again. I was holding sick call in the women's wing, when a young woman came to me with her arm supported and cradled in her top. I examined her and found that she had a broken humerus. (the upper arm bone) I asked her how this happened? She replied that she was on the top bunk, lost her balance and fell but her arm was trapped in the chain holding the bunk. She heard a snap and felt terrible pain, so she went on sick call. (TWO DAYS AGO) She had been going on sick call for two days and received Tylenol both times. I couldn't believe that the other nurses couldn't recognize a broken arm if it was staring them in the face. Not one of them even placed her on the list to see the doctor.

I called the night supervisor and informed her that I had an inmate with a broken arm, and she needed to be transported to the hospital. She refused my request and ordered me to place her on doctor's sick call the next morning. We argued back and forth for several minutes, but she refused to send the inmate to the hospital to have her arm set and casted.

The next day when I reported for work, I was summoned to the director's office and was told that I had errored in caring for the inmate. I was told that I should have overruled the nursing supervisor on duty, and sent the inmate to the hospital. I retorted that there was no provision in the rules to override a supervisor's order, and broached the subject that the nurses working for two days before me were so incompetent that they couldn't recognize a broken arm when the saw one. I knew what she was heading for, which was to get rid of me under any pretext that she could. I also recognized that she was so stupid that she had no counter argument for any point I made, and she was losing the argument entirely. The last thing the jail wanted was a nurse who was going to spot things, and point them out. That would force the sheriff to spend money to do something, and they never wanted to do that. If an inmate dies while in the jail the sheriff would investigate himself, some nurse would get fired, (usually the last one hired whether they were working or not) and things would go on as before. The girl with the broken arm never saw the doctor in the morning, the charges were dropped and she was released from the jail first thing to seek medical care on her own. I walked out that morning, and had another job by noon, and everyone was happy again.

The girl fell from the top bunk because the top bunk was visible from the men's barracks and the girls were able to communicate with their boyfriends by kneeling on the top bunk facing the window. They were crowded on the bunk, and she was pushed off by another inmate eager to take her place. She grabbed for the chain holding the bunk to break her fall, but her body weight twisting on the way down broke her arm.

GO AHEAD FIRE ME
Try to squeeze by each and every day

Very infrequently, nurses must deal with a patient complaint. Mine started innocently while passing meds in a patient's room. I was at the bedside assisting the female patient by pouring her water, when a female relative who was sitting at the bedside decided she needed answers to her questions. She asked me a pertinent question about the patient while I was in the room. I asker her who she was, and she reported that she was the daughter of the patient and the health care surrogate, so I answered her question. She then proceeded to ask several more and I answered those also.

Later in the shift the grapevine informed me that the visitor had made a complaint about me to the nursing office. I could expect to be called down to the office over it later in the day. Sure enough, after lunch I was summoned to report to the nursing office for a dressing down. When I arrived, there were three bigshots seated in the little office waiting for me.

I was told that the daughter of the patient had made a complaint that I had said things in the room that she didn't want her mother to hear. (are you bullshitting me) If the daughter did not want the mother to hear something, she had two options. The first was to follow me out of the room and ask me in the hallway where the mother could not hear the answer, or second, don't ask the question in the patient's room in front of the mother. And there was a third alternative, ask the doctor.

Of course, the big shots tried to make me out to be wrong, but the relative had made the error and refused to take responsibility for it. I couldn't understand why nursing big shots could not see what had happened and forget it, but they never did.

At this point it is probably instructive to typify the standard nurse executive, officer, boss, or big shot.

When they were hired as a boss, they were placed on a scale and if they were over 250 lbs. they were hired.

If they had a dirty lab coat with wads of papers in the pocket they were hired.

If the lab coat had a torn pocket from being over full, they were hired.

If their feet hurt when they walked and they waddled down the hallway they were hired.

If the sides were broken out of their shoes, they were hired

If their body was so big it made their head look little, they were hired.

If they liked to sit in an office as big as a broom closet, they were hired.

If they liked to tell you how to do your job, but couldn't do it themselves, they were hired.

If they spent more time in the cafeteria than on the unit, they were hired.

I think you get the idea, they were not usually looked up to by the staff. In fact, most of the staff I knew could function better if the big shot was absent, or gone entirely. Which brings me to the next story.

I was working telemetry with an exhausting patient load of six desperately ill patients. Each one could and should have had 1 to 1 nursing, this was typical of the assignments male nurses got on the floor. We always got the heaviest load just because we were men. One of the patients I had just received from surgical ICU. He had a cranial bleed and 50% of his brain was removed along with half of his skull. He was comatose but alive and was in terrible shape. He had been in ICU for over a week and had ulcers all over his posterior surfaces. There were decubitus (ulcers) on the back of his head, his coccyx, and both heels (so much for 1 to 1 care) He required full care and had to be rolled every two hours, minimum. He also was sweaty and smelled having received no attention for the entire time in ICU. The next was on six different IV solutions requiring two IV poles to hang them from. The next was a quad requiring total care, and so on for the other three. It was a crushing load of patients for anyone. I had been working for about nine hours under this load, and was over an hour behind on my meds when I was approached by the charge nurse with a summons to the nursing office. I had three more hours to work and was trying my upmost to get my meds in line with the times, and answer all the lights, and process all the orders that a group of physicians had written. I had no time for the bullshit I was confronted with at the nursing office. I told the charge nurse that I was not going down. I gave no explanation because she could see me working like a dog. Fifteen minutes later she said that they were waiting for me and I had better get down to the office right now. At that point I told her that she knew my response, so she walked away. Five minutes later she said that they were sending a nurse up to replace me so I could go down stairs. That was a joke indeed. They sent up a new nurse just out of school so I took her to the first room while I hung IV bags and explained to the what was going on with that patient. We went to the second room and I was explaining the problems there when she asked me if I also had the quad in the next bed, and I said yes. She turned on her heel and walked out, I never saw her again so I continued on with my work. I learned later that she reported to the bosses that she refused the assignment and that they would have to send at least two nurses for that load of patients. I continued to refuse to go down stairs until after the shift was over and I had given report to the next nurse. By then my load was broken up between three other nurses each receiving one or two of my patients. I then went to the nursing office where two bosses were still sitting waiting. They informed me that they had been there for almost four hours waiting for me. Both sore and very tired I asked them immediately if they intended to fire me on the spot or not. They said there was no intention to fire me during this meeting. I said "good, if you change your mind call me at home" and walked out of the office and went home. I was not fired, and the meeting never took place, I never knew what they wanted but was sure it was about the problem I had heard about, but was too tired to care. Both the supervisors and I knew that I could have another job in an hour at another hospital. They were already trying to run a telemetry unit with only two qualified telemetry nurses, the rest were not trained and never wanted to be. The other tele nurse was an LPN, so I was the only credentialed RN working that shift so they were screwed if they fired me. This is typical of most hospitals in Florida. They want to keep payroll to a minimum, so they hire the newest most inexperienced nurses they can get, and try to squeeze by each and every day hoping the bottom won't fall out, but it does, often. Deaths occur that could have been avoided if the nurses were on the ball and recognized problems quickly before the patient became critical and moved beyond the point where they could be recovered.

RICHARD

I got Richard to help a little

I was working for a corporate nursing agency, they supplied nurses to fill-in vacancies at only hospitals they owned. I was called and asked if I would work outside the county if they gave me a bonus to do it. I agreed, and received the assignment to drive a good distance to fill in for a large group of staff nurses who quit as a group because of poor working conditions and low pay.

I arrived at the hospital, and while walking to the building, I encountered several RN's that I had worked with in the past also walking from the parking lot. We had all been drafted to fill in vacant shift positions. One of the nurses Richard and I were assigned to the telemetry unit together. We began our shift and were assigned a very large group of patients to take care of. I asked the charge RN, why the extra patients, and she responded that we were the only RN's they could get, we were it. As usual, I went to work, and began seeing to my patients. It was not long before my med pass was behind, and I was trying to grind through the shift. I noticed that Richard was in the nurses lounge reading. I hurried in, and asked him how in the hell he could find the time to sit and read. He said, "I flushed the meds down the toilet." I almost crapped myself, he actually meant it. He said that he gave the essential meds, but all the other stuff like vitamins, stomach meds, specialty stuff were all flushed. He said that this hospital was going to get what they paid for, he was not going to kill himself because they were short handed, it was their problem not his. I almost fell over, but went back to work doing the right thing.

I was alerted by the monitor tech that a patient was showing cardiac problems on the monitor, and I needed to check on them right away. I went to the room, and sure enough the wall monitor showed a serious issue developing. I reviewed the meds, and there were orders for a special IV drip to be started to arrest the problem. I immediately started the drip, but was having issued with his response to the medication, I thought he needed additional orders, and a transfer to CCU right away.

I went to the charge RN and reported the problem, and was told that CCU was short nurses, and there was no way to transfer the patient there in the immediate future. I told the RN to call 911 and have the patient transferred to a hospital that could take the patient into their CCU. She refused, and said that I would have to take care of the patient until the end of my shift, and then she would see what the oncoming charge wanted to do. I told her to assume the care of this patient so I could see to my other patients, and she refused. I further told her that if the patient died on my shift I would call the police and have her charged with murder. At that point she started calling administrators, and any one else she could get in touch with, saying I had threatened her.

I returned to care for the patient, and did 1/1 nursing until the end of the shift, but the patient vacillated between stable and unstable continuously. I got Richard to help a little, but this kind of stuff was bullshit. Now I knew why the staff nurses quit as a group, and I followed their example and did the same. Richard worked there another month and he quit too.

A quick note on Richard:

The first time I came across him was working 3-11 shift at a local hospital. Richard followed me on the same unit but the 11-7 shift. He was a Martinet, a person who was constantly picking at other nurses work, and tattling on every little thing. For the most part he was hated by the nurses on the 3-11 shift for that reason, always telling tales. Richard liked 11-7 shift because for the most part it was easier to work 11-7, and he liked easy. On this occasion, he was ratting on me, and I was getting really tired of it. I decided to get even with him in a big way. Before the end of my shift I gave every patient prune juice, and warm apple juice to drink. I gave report to Richard and left for the night, and he took over. When I came in at 3 o'clock every patient told me what a great BM they had last evening, and they were all smiling, and very happy and satisfied. One even reported that he thought it was the best BM he had ever had. At 11 o'clock a bedraggled Richard showed his face, and he was not himself. He approached me and asked me what I had done to make all the patients shit their brains out all night long. He told me that he ran out of linen and had to go to two other floors to get enough linen to change all the messed beds. He said that he never worked that hard since he became an RN. I then told him about his little tattling on me all the time, and if he tattled again, he would have another explosive night to deal with. We reach a truce that night, and went on to work together on several other assignments, from private duty, to agency work and others with no problems again.

TAKE YOUR SEATS, OPEN YOUR BOOKS
Was I to experience the same result with every problem student?

I took a job as a clinical and didactic instructor at a local college. This school was educating both RN's and LPN's. I was hired into the LPN program, and was responsible for the last year of training, and to get the class through the national LPN exam with a passing grade.

The exam was graded on a national basis with the median score being the passing grade nationally. At the time I began teaching, I believe the passing mark was 78.9. If a nursing schools average falls below that mark the school is placed on probation. If the grades on the very next exam do not improve, the school is dropped from the program and is essentially out of business.

At the time of my hire the school was tip toeing on the edge of probation with the last graduating class. I had my work cut out for me, as the school was having trouble keeping competent instructors employed. Instructor after instructor had either quit or been fired, some in the middle of the class term. The next class was in an uproar sweating the exam without a decent instructor to guide them through this tough time.

Additionally, there were separate clinical instructors who went to outside locations to supervise the students in their work experiences. The classroom instructor (professor) controlled all of the outside clinical people, and was responsible for all their work with the students. The professor was also responsible for drawing up the lesson plans and formulating and giving the exams. The overall semester work plan was produced by the college, which covered every subject necessary in the LPN curriculum, which was used as a basis for all lesson plans. There was significant latitude given to the instructor to add quality instruction based on guidelines in the curriculum. I began instructing midway through the first semester in a two semester final year, because the instructor had quit midterm. I was tasked with raising the class marks, and taking over one of the clinical instructor jobs also, since there were more than twelve students in the class. I had to use an additional clinical instructor because no clinical instructor can supervise more than twelve students in work experience, that is the maximum.

The students were a motley crew of mostly women, one transvestite, and a few men. I found them moderately motivated, with one really bad slacker in the group which was trouble on the hoof. How she had gotten to the senior year in school, I had no idea. (I would find out soon enough) I had not taught very long when the slacker was missing from the classroom more than she was present in the first weeks. Students are allowed three absences during the semester or they are dropped from the program, and she used the three right away. The first exam I gave, I caught her cheating, and sent her before the disciplinary board. She was able to talk her way out of her dilemma and continued in the class. I had only one more exam to give in the semester and she got the lowest mark in the class, but barely squeaked through.

After the disciplinary board experience, I went to the dean of the school and reported that the slacker was an unacceptable student, would make a horrible nurse, and had no business being in nursing school. The dean informed me that the slacker was given a passing grade by the disciplinary committee for the exam she cheated on because the plan was to fail her in the last semester of the senior year. She would never get to graduate, and the school would get paid the full amount. I also found out that her church was footing the bill for her education. Now I understood why she was so lax in pursuit of a nursing license. Since I had no prior experience with the school or the students, I played my role, and the student was unable to pass any exam in the last semester and flunked out. Overall, the class scored 99% on the licensure exam, and the school was out of trouble, and I was happy.

During the next two years there were no problems with

students or the instruction. I was flying high with several 100% classes. I received the next class and began as before with classroom and clinical instruction in the first semester. Several students were moved on to me that had barely made it through the last semester with poor test grades. I saw this as a big problem, so I began to tutor them before class to help them to get in line with the rest of the class. The marginal students by this time were well integrated into the class with friends they went through clinicals with. One quit after flunking the first test, and the second flunked the test, but wanted to keep trying. She went through the semester in trouble all the way and unfortunately, went down hard on the final exam. Unfortunately, she had flunked out of school. I had already told her that she should repeat the semester, and with the additional instruction she would probably pass and get to take the licensure exam. The student angrily refused my counseling and tried another route. She went to a meeting she had arranged with the dean and stated that she was sure she could do the work and wanted another chance. I had no knowledge of her visit with the dean, and was caught by surprise when I found out what had transpired during the visit. The dean asked for her final exam to be brought to her office, and began to invalidate questions on the exam, just enough to get the student through the semester into the next year.

When I found out what had happened, I refused to sign her transcript, and evaluation, and test, as prescribed by the school, and protested the test score changes to the dean. I was told by the second in command that, "on the dean's orders she was passed through, and I was to fail her in the final semester." Again, the school would get the full tuition and the student would be failed at the end of the final year. Since I had remembered the first semester of my employment when the same thing was told to me, I rebelled. Was I to experience this same result with every problem student that had managed to slip through into my final classes?

Since money seemed to be the only thing that the dean cared about, I would not let her collect the last semesters money, or if she did get the money, I would take it away from her in another way. First, I insisted on a pay raise equivalent to the tuition. Second, if she rebuffed the raise, I would quit and force her to hire both a clinical instructor, and classroom instructor which would cost her more. Third, she would lose the 100% licensure exam pass rate which she enjoyed for the last two years.

The dean rebuffed my pay raise option which I fully expected her to do. She understood that I was punishing her for screwing with the test marks, but that was her method of keeping the cash flow coming in. I knew she was in a bad position but she was going to take her chances going back to the old hire and fire routine she had done before when her test scores on the national exam were marginal. As I had done my entire career, I had another job two days later and gave my notice. The dean sent her second in command to talk to me asking if I could teach a little while longer, hoping this would blow over, but I stuck to my exit date. Eventually the school found someone to replace me on the classroom and clinical sites, but were never again able to attain the scores on the national exam that I had achieved. Unknown to the school or other instructors, I had stumbled onto a formula for passing the licensure exam that worked. It was a simple thing, but it worked like a charm on every student who tried it. Word got around among the students that if they got into my class, they would get a license, so there was always keen interest to get into my class. I enjoyed instructing, but I would not participate in the scheme to bilk the students out of their tuition, and deny them the license they had paid for.

GOLFERS

The golfers legs were under the cart

In Florida, golf is a popular sport, especially among the elderly. As a sport, it is not noted for injuries, but they happen frequently. I have had patients who had heart attacks while playing golf and suffered other injuries. In fact, the first dead person I saw was rushed into the E.R. via ambulance after having a heart attack while playing the game. He expired shortly after arriving at the hospital. Another patient I had, drove himself from the course to the E.R. While he was playing the 9th hole he experienced chest pain. Well a little angina was not going to stop him. Before coming to the hospital, he finished playing the back nine. Based on an EKG and labs, the E.R. doctor diagnosed a heart attack. The patient was rushed into the cath lab and cardiac stents were placed.

One patient I took care of was a seventy-five year old female who had both of her legs broken while playing golf. What happened was, she got of the golf cart to hit her ball. The ball was next to the cart, so to get a good swing at the ball she asked her girlfriend who was in the cart to move the cart forward. Instead of putting cart in drive, her friend put it into reverse with the wheels turned and ran the woman over. The golfer's legs were under the cart between the front and back wheels. The golfer was screaming in pain. Her friend panicked and put the cart in drive and ran over the golfer a second time.

Another patient I had (a seventy-eight year old male) was made C.M.O. (comfort measures only) and was transferred to hospice as a result of a golfing mishap. The man was attempting to get into his golf cart when he tripped and hit his head against the windshield post of the cart. The fall resulted in a concussion and he was brought to the hospital. He spent two days in the hospital, and was transferred to a rehab. He was supposed to spend five days in rehab, and then be discharged to home. After three days in rehab, he was back in the hospital. Besides a concussion, the man had an enlarged prostate. At the rehab, nobody was monitoring his urinary output. He never emptied his bladder, thus urine backed up into his kidneys. As a result, he developed a urinary tract infection and renal insufficiency. Urinary tract infections can be devastating to an elderly patient, often causing mental confusion. This patient became very lethargic and would not eat, so a feeding tube was inserted through his nose into the stomach. To ensure his urinary output was sufficient a urinary catheter was inserted into the bladder. A central line was placed because the infectious disease doctor believed he needed to be on long term antibiotics.

After several days of hospitalization, no improvement was shown, so the wife and the doctors decided to suspend all treatment and make him comfort measures only (C.M.O.). He was then transferred to hospice. Just think, before his golfing accident he was an active senior; golfing, driving his car, going out to dinner and shopping.

From living next to a golf course, I can tell you one thing elderly male golfers like to do is driving their golf carts fast. I had a seventy year out patient who tipped his cart over while making a sharp turn at break neck speed. This resulted in a broken hip, four days in the hospital, and then discharged to home with home health care. You would think he would have realized that a golf cart is not aerodynamically designed and sharp turns should not be made at maximum speed.

THE GREATEST GENERATION

She was something of a curiosity with the younger nurses

Working 3-11 shift in a local hospital, we from time to time received elderly patients with a tattooed number on their forearm. These patients were European concentration camp survivors. In this case, it was an elderly Polish woman suffering from an end of life illness. Her tattoo was tough to read because she had tried to cover it up by having a flesh color tattoo placed over it on her arm. We did not ask her about her experience because trying to cover it up meant that she probably didn't want to discuss it. She was a very pleasant old lady, and word spread about her unfortunate experience, so, many nurses came in to see her, and to see the tattoo without being obvious, she was something of a curiosity with the younger nurses who had never seen someone like her. She enjoyed meeting all the visitors, it made her days pass quickly.

The old lady found that she did not like hospital food, and she was preoccupied with getting sausages one night for supper. She had this craving, so I decided to leave a note in the doctor's section of the chart to have the attending physician order sausages for her to eat, since she wanted them so badly.

The next evening when I came to work, a young doctor was in her room talking to her. The young doctor was covering for her attending physician. I listened to what he was saying as I stood by the door of the room. He was telling the old woman how bad sausages were for her, how they oozed fat, they were filled with all kinds of mystery meat, etc. After he finished, he told her that in good conscience, he could not order sausages for her to eat. I almost fell over when I heard that. Here was a concentration camp survivor, dying in a local hospital, who wanted sausages for one of her last meals, and the doctor was worried about her intake of cholesterol, are you bullshitting me!!!!!

The next day the old woman was transferred to Hospice to live out her last few days, and I hope someone gave her the sausages to eat.

The next patient I received was a direct admission that came from a doctor's office. It was a gentleman in his eighties suffering from congestive heart failure (meaning that his heart was unable to move around enough fluid to prevent a buildup in the lungs) He had received a dose of diuretic at the doctor's office, but was still in some distress. Along with the patient came a sheet of orders to be accomplished on the floor where I was assigned. I reviewed the orders, and before I completed the full admission, I gave him an injection of diuretic to follow up on his initial dose given by his family physician. I inserted an IV, and a Foley catheter into his bladder to drain his bladder of fluid.

After an hour he was resting comfortably, so I completed the admission process. The gentleman spoke with a German accent, and owned a specialty machine shop in the community near the hospital. The next day I had an opportunity to talk with the man and found out that he had been in WW 2 and fought on the German side. He was a graduate of one of the German military academies called the Kriegsschule, and the tank school called the Panzertruppenschule. He fought on the western front against the Russians. He was a tank commander, and during one of the battles in Russia his tank was disabled. Both he and one crewman were able to exit the tank through an escape hatch in the bottom of the tank. Being on foot during the battle he started making his way back to German lines, when he came upon the rear of the Russian attacking force. He was spotted, and subsequently captured, where he was taken to a local home where two other German soldiers were being held. They were all in the large main room of the house and were seated at a large table on an attached heavy bench. In order to assure that the prisoners would not try to escape, their hands were nailed to the large heavy table. The Russians left and continued advancing on the German front lines. Being the only officer, he resolved not to be there when the Russians returned, so he stood up and ripped his hands loose from the nails through his hands causing severe damage to his hands. He exited the cottage and secured a hiding place until dark. After dark he carefully made his way back to the German lines alone. Once he was taken to the German aid station, the extent of damage to his hands was evident, and he was loaded onto a small aircraft used for the purpose of removing injured officers and men back to Germany for treatment. The aircraft were landed on the battlefield to extricate cases for advanced treatment at the closest German held hospital. In his case he was flown back to a suburb of Berlin to have hand surgery. He had numerous surgeries, and was still in the recovery section of the hospital when it was overrun by the American Army. Since he was not a Nazi party member, and was a qualified machinist he was considered for immigration to the US after his discharge from the German Army. He settled in Florida and married a local woman from a German family he met at a local party. He worked at a machine shop until his employer helped set him up in business doing specialty jobs that the big shop couldn't handle. The gentleman was in the hospital for a week, and was discharged on new medication to keep from a repeat of his CHF, I never saw him again, and yes, his hands were a mass of scar tissue but they functioned well enough for him to do his job.

THE SINGER

I tried to make it sound like the Beach Boys song

This story is about the Beach Boy's song "Help Me Rhonda", a nurse named Rhonda, and an identical twin who was a doctor.

Let's start with the doctor, she was in her late forty's early fifties, she was an internal medicine doctor who had graduated from medical school in Poland. Both her and her identical twin sister were Polish physicians who emigrated to the United States, and were both able to pass the Medical Practice exam taken by foreign trained doctors to allow them to practice medicine in the US.

The RN named Rhonda was a PRN (worked as needed) nurse who from time to time worked with me when a staff nurse was absent.

I was working 3-11 shift at a local hospital, and Rhonda was working adjacent in the same hallway with me. I had worked with her many times in the past, and she was great to work with, always jovial, and very competent. When I needed another RN to help me pull a patient up in the bed, I would go to the door of the room, and signal that I needed help. If Rhonda was working I would call "Help me Rhonda, Help, Help, me Rhonda" to get her attention, and I tried to make it sound like the Beach Boy's song.

On this night, we were finishing up our shift, and were both writing our notes at stations next to each other, and the doctor was at a third station on the other side of me, we were all writing. I thought it was a good time to burst into song, so I started singing, "Help me Rhonda, Help Help me Rhonda, Help me Rhonda, Get Her out of my Heart." Rhonda looked up from her notes with a big smile on her face, and said "don't quit your day job." When suddenly the doctor next to me looked up talking to Rhonda and said, "Oh, I didn't think he was so bad." With that, we all broke out laughing for a few minutes, and then we all went back to work again finishing our notes.

CONVERSATION

Very interesting patients and their Stories

The best part of my job is, I get to talk to interesting patients. As a nurse I have taken care of many interesting people such as; the judge who presided over the Sam Sheppard murder trial, a former assistant sergeant at arms of the U.S. Senate (he knew Jack Kennedy and Lyndon Johnson), a secret service agent who protected the Nixon girls, another secret service agent who protected Richard Nixon and still another agent who protected foreign dignitaries that were visiting the U.S., a baseball hall of fame inductee, a famous professional wrestler, a U.S. congressman, a former high ranking diplomat, Al Capone's lawyer, a retired Marine Corps colonel who used to go shooting with Al Capone's brother and other patients who are too numerous to mention.

I like talking to these patients because they often present a narrative that is at odds with the media and academia. I am particularly fascinated by veterans. I have not only taken care of American veterans, but also men who had served in the Canadian, British, Polish and German armed forces. There two former German soldiers I will not forget. The first was a medic from Lithuania. I asked him "how did a Lithuanian end up in the Germany army"? His response was "I got drafted." He went on to explain that in 1941 the Germans invaded Lithuania and in 1943 he got drafted into the German Army. He explained when the war ended his division was in Czechoslovakia. He told me his division tried to surrender to the Americans, but the Americans told them they could not accept any more Germans prisoners, so they waited for three days for the Red Army to show up. He told me the Americans had tanks, trucks and jeeps. The Soviets had ox carts. After he surrendered, he spent ten years in a Soviet prison camp before being released. Upon being released, he was returned to Germany. He told me that a lot of German soldiers died in captivity.

The other former German soldier I took care of had been a 1st lieutenant in a tank unit. He had been at Stalingrad and refused to surrender with the rest of the German forces. He explained to me he just drove his tank through Soviet lines. For some reason, the Soviets thought his tank was a Red Army tank and allowed it to pass. He eventually drove through the Soviet encirclement and reached German lines. I asked him what he thought of the quality of the Italian, Hungarian and Rumanian troops (Germany's allies on the Eastern Front). I told him that we were led to believe that the troops from these nations were really lousy soldiers. He responded that was not the case.

He told me that the soldiers from these countries were very religious. When the Soviets attacked, they would place women in the front of their advancing troops. The Italians, Hungarians and Rumanians refused to shoot women. When the war ended, he surrendered to the Canadian Army and was treated well. After being release from a P.O.W. camp, he went to work for a multinational company as an engineer. His work took him to Africa because, he told me his company was interested in both cheap sources of labor and the bottom line.

Another patient who I found interesting was Joe, a Jewish-American veteran from Savannah Georgia. One does not think of American Jews and Savannah, but this veteran told me that Savannah was home to one of the earliest Jewish communities in the U.S. Joe said his family had lived in Savannah for over 250 years. He told me his grandmother remembers the city's occupation by Union troops. I asked him if the there was widespread looting by Union soldiers when Savannah fell. According to his grandmother most of the Union soldiers behaved well, some Union troops engaged in robbing civilians, but this was done by stragglers (his grandmother called them ragamuffins) who followed the main body of Sherman's army.

I asked Joe about his military service. In 1933 he joined a cavalry unit in the Georgia National Guard, in order to pick up girls. Joe told me he thought it would be glamorous riding a horse wearing a dress uniform (back then the cavalry had horses) and thus girls would be attracted to him. He said in 1940 the Georgia National guard was federalized and their horses were taken away replaced by trucks. He ended up in North Africa where he was captured by the Germans.

I asked him how that happened. He told me one night his battalion received orders to pull back. Those orders were never communicated to his company, so the company to the right and the one to the left of his company withdrew. In the morning his company was surrounded by Germans, so they surrendered. He told me he was treated very well by the Germans. They congratulated him on being a prisoner. By being a prisoner, he was guaranteed, to survive the war. When the German Army departed from North Africa they left behind their American prisoners. His prison camp was liberated by the American Army.

He took part in the invasion of Italy. While fighting in Italy, he was severely wounded. He was evacuated to a military hospital in Jacksonville Florida. After recovering from his wounds, he was placed in charge of the hospital ambulances. When the war ended, he was discharged with the rank of master sergeant. He looked to me like the kind of senior N.C.O. that any officer would be thrilled to have. He was experienced, level headed and practical.

Another veteran who story I found interesting was a former paratrooper who took part in the liberation of Corregidor. He told me that his company jumped at 300 feet over the island. This was an extremely low jump and resulted in half of his company being injured. He suffered a sprained ankle. During the fighting he and two other paratroopers found a stash of Japanese sake. That night he and his two friends got drunk and slept through a Japanese bonsai attack on a neighboring company.

INSISTENCE

The Squeaky Wheel Gets Government Benefits

After graduating from L.P.N. school, my first job was working at a V.A. nursing home. The care given at that nursing home was outstanding. I refer to it as the Cadillac of nursing homes. The place was immaculate. Not a single patient had a bed sore. All the patients were up, out of bed, and in the dinning room for meals. The woman who ran the nursing home was a well dressed, well spoken, no nonsense Black woman. Except for me, all the nurses and aides were long time V.A. employees, who were close to retirement. The work was routine, so it was a great place to spend a few years before retirement.

Unfortunately the near by V.A. hospital had less than a stellar reputation. One day we received a patient from the hospital. He was a recent bilateral above the knee amputee. In my thirty-eight years in nursing, I have never seen anything that was done to this man. It was beyond malpractice, it was an atrocity. Bones were sticking through the stumps of his legs. We used Neosporin on a 2x2 to cover the bones. For pain the patient had plain Tylenol. The patient was in constant pain. When the nurse practitioner who covered the nursing home saw the patient she was livid. She could not believe only Tylenol was ordered for this man's pain. She immediate wrote for morphine.

As I spent more time working with the man, I got to know his background. He joined the army at the tail end of World War II. When the war ended he went into the army reserve. When the Korean War broke out he was put on active duty and sent to Korea. While serving in Korea he got a severe case of frostbit on his lower legs and feet. He returned home and was discharged from the army. After his discharge, he got a job driving a truck from the orange groves to the processing plant. During his time working as a truck driver, he suffered from poor circulation in his legs and feet, and neuropathy. He applied to the V.A. for disability, but was denied. The government said his circulatory problem were not due to frostbit, but were caused by his driving a truck. The V.A. did agree to amputate his legs for free. The patient and his family were rural Southerners. These people are the type of people who complain.

At the same time I had another patient a retiree from N.Y., who was morbidly obese and suffered from a stroke. While he was in the nursing home getting rehab, his family applied for him to get a van with the controls in the steering wheel. The V.A. will provide a veteran who can not use his legs a van with braking and gas controls in the steering wheel, if his disability was service related. The V.A. turned the New Yorker down. They said his stroke was not service related because it occurred thirty-nine years after he was discharged from the army. Well his family started calling up their congressman and senator. To make a long story short the New Yorker got the van and the Southerner got a botch operation.

WHAT ABOUT MY HUSBAND?

A second opportunity to give your life for your country

The V.A. had a respite program for the care givers of disabled. If a family member was taking care of a disabled veteran at home every six months they were allowed to bring the veteran into a V.A. nursing home for two weeks. This gives the care giver a much needed break   One day we got such a patient at the nursing home. He was dropped in front of the nursing station and the care giver left before I could meet her. The man was in his early fifties, his clothes looked like they came from the Salvation Army dumpster, he was sitting on a filthy wheelchair and he stunk. He also suffered from late onset diabetes and his blood sugar was elevated.

The first thing I did to put on gloves and a gown.   I wanted to make sure I didn't catch anything from the patient. I have known nurses who have gotten scabies from patients and on one occasion I knew a nurse whose dog got C-Diff (an infection that causes among other things loose stools) by licking her shoes. Next was to get him out of his dirty clothes and put him on a shower chair. I rolled the vet into the shower and literally hosed him off. This would not be the last time I would hose off a new patient. Later when worked at large community hospital, I would frequently have to do this to homeless patients. After being cleaned, I dressed him in V.A. pajamas. After the shower, I cleaned his wheelchair.

Over the next three days, the patient seemed to be doing well. On the fourth day, a diabetic ulcer opened up on his foot. The nurse practitioner, assigned to the nursing home, decided to move the patient to the hospital.

Three days after we moved him to the hospital an attractive well dressed woman in her mid forties showed up at the nursing home wanting to know what I did to her husband.

She said "when I left him here he was in good shape." She mentioned her husband's name, but it did not register. I stood there totally flabbergasted. Finally, the ward clerk seeing my confusion pulled me aside and said "you know the man that stunk." Then I realized what she was talking about. I explained to her all I did was clean her husband and get his blood sugar under control. When a sore developed on his foot the nurse practitioner decided to move him to the hospital. She told the nurse practitioner that "if he dies the V.A. disability checks will stop" and she will have to go to work for a living. I did not, but I felt like telling her to join the rest of us that who are working for a living. It was evident to me the wife was providing her husband with a bare minimum of care and viewed him as a cash cow.

Later I discussed the situation with older V.A. nurses. They explained to me what I encountered was not unique. It was not usual for family members to live off a veteran's disability check. The veteran would receive almost none of the money from their check. I was told about a Vietnam War vet whose parents took most of his disability check for their own expenses. They drove a Cadillac and they did not give their son enough money to buy socks. The nurses bought the guy socks. I thought there must be a special place in hell for those who take advantage of the disabled.

I do not know what happened to my patient. I never saw him or his wife again. My guess he was probably discharged from the V.A. hospital. I hope they did not amputate his foot. There is some truth in the old adage "the V.A. gives you a second opportunity to give your life for your country."

NOT A QUITTER

I informed her I would take my chances

Attending nursing school taught me many things, the first was sit in class and don't say a thing. Nursing instructors like to be right all the time, and if you think they are wrong, you had better keep your big mouth shut. I was in my second year of nursing school when we had a class on A.I.D.S. and it didn't go well. The instructor was describing how the disease was going to go from the gay community into the general population and become a pandemic. I took issue with her position, and she didn't like it at all. I made a rational argument against her position, and she got nasty because she had never been challenged before. She vowed to get even when I submitted my 20 page term paper to her to be marked.

I submitted the paper, and she took her revenge by marking a 60 on the paper. (I had never received less than a 98 before) I was called in and more or less ordered to drop out of the school, and repeat the semester because of the low mark. She reported that I needed an 80 on the final exam, and I had not received an 80 on a final exam since I had been in the school. (I was attending school at night and working 60 hrs. a week at my job) I refused to quit, and informed her I would take my chances with the test. She didn't retort, so I left her office and told her I would never quit at anything, and I wouldn't start now. After I took the exam I waited for my mark, and was at work when I received a call from the school. It was the instructor on the line and she informed me that I received an 82 on the final exam. I never had to deal with her again, and graduated on time.

SIDE JOBS

I was not going to wind up in the hospital over an $8.00 tip

Many times side jobs are more interesting and more fun than the full time job which pays the bills. In this case I took a part time job where I did not have to get dirty and wore a suit and tie, and drove nice shiny Cadillacs. It was working for a livery outfit. Livery is a garage full of Cadillacs that lease them to funeral directors, and provides the drivers for the equipment too. The position entails picking up the car at the garage, going to a home somewhere in the area, and taking a family to the funeral home for the service. During the service you wait in the embalming room for the service to be over, and on the signal, bring the car around to the front of the building to collect the family. From the funeral home, you either go to a church, or the cemetery for the burial, and then drive the family home.

In this experience I was hired to take a hearse to a cemetery for exhumation of an old Italian man who had died ten years before. He was being dug up to be sent back home to Italy to be reburied. His family was footing the bill for the entire cost which was extensive. A back hoe dug down to the concrete rough box, and hauled the heavy lid off of the vault in the grave. The vault was filled with wet mud up to the top. Cemetery workers shoveled the dirt out of the vault until the coffin was seen. The straps were found and attached to the back hoe and the coffin was pulled out of the wet vault leaving behind water and mud. The coffin was swung into the hears, and taken back to the rear street of the funeral palor. There the coffin was unloaded by eight men, and opened and turned on its side. The coffin was filled with wet mud that had seeped inside over the time it had been buried. A hose was used to wash the dirt out of the coffin until the old Italian man was located. He was pulled from the wet mud in the coffin and after being hosed off we picked him up and placed him in a specially purchased grey travel coffin similar to the one JFK was placed in for his trip from Dallas. In picking up the old man it was like handling a statue, he was as solid as one. The travel coffin was then closed, and then plaCed back into the hearse for the trip to the airport.

If a livery driver is used as a pallbearer, he gets a set amount for his services in addition to the salary for driving the limo. In this case one other driver and I were called upon to serve as pallbearers. The family had decided that they wanted the grandchildren to carry the casket, so we were augmenting their job. The only problem was that the grandchildren were a bunch of kids some as young as 10 years old. This was madness because a body can weigh over 250 lbs. plus the weight of the coffin. There is no way two men and a bunch of kids can haul the coffin through the cemetery to the grave. We managed to get the coffin off the trolley (used to remove the coffin from the funeral home to the hearse) into the hearse because the action was just sliding the casket onto the rollers in the cargo area of the hearse. At the church we did the same thing in reverse so that was OK. The problem arose when we got to the cemetery and the trek to the grave was a 50 yard up hill struggle from the road where the hearse was parked. A trolley can't be used up hill over grass, the coffin had to be carried, or more realistically lugged by a group of strong men up to the job. I knew we were in big trouble when I again saw the inexperienced group of kids line up to carry. The other man was on the head on the right side and I was on the left foot, and the kids were interspersed between us, it was madness. We retracted the coffin from the hearse and I felt the full weight of the coffin and judged it to be in the neighborhood of 300 lbs. or so. That meant that the two of us would have 150 lbs. each, and going up a steep hill the inertia and tilt of the coffin would drop most of the weight to me on the back of the box. I think I made it about four or five steps, and decided to let the little kids feel the weight because I couldn't carry it the 50 yards up hill. When the funeral director saw the coffin corner dropping toward the ground, he moved up and grabbed the back of the coffin trying to pick it up and get it back into position. I heard him groaning, and grunting while trying to advance with the weight of the box bending him over more and more as we advanced up the hill. The more he struggled, the more weight I let him carry until by the time we reached the graveside he was spent. After we lowered the casket onto the elevator at the graveside, he got me on the side and told me that he was not going to pay me for being a pallbearer. I told him I could care less, kids can't carry a coffin and I hope you learned something. He was pissed, but I was not going to wind up in the hospital over an $8.00 tip.

One of the funeral directors I helped out used to have a connection in the medical examiner's office who contacted him after they were finished with an unclaimed body. I would take it to a crematorium and have it cremated. The ashes were mailed to the funeral home to be stored until or if someone wanted to claim them. A couple of boxes arrived one day and I had no place to put them as the shelves in the embalming room were full. I asked the director where he wanted them placed since the shelves were full, and there was a whole wall of shelves with dozens of boxes on them. He said to just make room for them, so I took off two older boxes, and threw them in the trash and replaced them with the two new boxes. They kept coming, and I kept making room.

You hear stories about hair and fingernails growing after death, about bodies sitting up in the morgue. As a novice in the funeral business, I asked all these questions of an embalmer. He told me that when he was through with a body, he guaranteed me it was never going to sit up ever. And the hair and fingernail story was total bullshit too. One day a truck dropped off a wooden casket like the ones used in the old west. It was painted with gloss white enamel, and hand lettered in a crude way on the lid "From the Funeral Homes of Zambia." It was a pilot who had crashed his bush plane and was burned in the crash. We pried off the lid of the coffin expecting to find a body, but all we found was a thin sheet of lead soldered onto a lead lined coffin. There was a plumber working there, so he was enlisted to melt the solder and peel back the lead seal. When it was pulled back, there was the corpse still in the sitting position with his hands still on a non-existing steering yoke of the plane, he was frozen in time burned to a crisp in position. A coffin had been selected by the family, so it was wheeled into position, and the body was pulled from the coffin and placed into the newly purchased casket for the closed casket ceremony upstairs. The Zambia coffin was hosed out on the back street and the plumber took it away to salvage the scrap lead lining the coffin.

One day a group of Jewish men arrived to treat a body that was not being embalmed. They wore wide brimmed black hats and black clothing, one of them was disheveled and somewhat dirty looking in a black raincoat. The body was on the porcelain embalming table awaiting the men. Two of them set to work chanting while they mixed something with water in a couple of buckets they brought in with them. After several minutes they motioned to the dirty looking guy, who incidentally, was much younger than the other two, to get into position. He walked to the head of the table, fastened his raincoat collar shut, sat the body up from behind and held it there. The other two proceeded to slosh the buckets full of solution up the front of the body, over the shoulders and head, and onto the poor young guy holding the body up. His hat was soaked dripping off the brim onto his shoulders, while he sputtered and spit out what had gone onto his lips. He was soaked which explained his condition when he came in the door of the embalming room. When the two sloshers finished, they all packed up their buckets and solution and left. We dressed the body in a white bag called a shroud and placed him into a simple wooden coffin. It was a case where there was 24 hours to bury the patient in the ground, so he was taken away immediately when the washing was done.

This was a 2 limo job in a wealthy suburb of the city. The home was surrounded with hedges over 10 ft. tall with a semicircular driveway in front of a large stone colonial home. We pulled up in front of the home, and before we could knock, a large group of people exited the home and made for the open limousine doors. We had jump seats (folding seats in front of the rear seats) so we could take everyone that came out. The funeral was for the owner of a popular label of women's blouses and leisure clothing, and the people in the limo's were his family. We transported them to the funeral home where the service was held, and to the cemetery, and back home again. When we entered the circular driveway, I felt a strange cold breeze on my head and neck before the vehicle had stopped. I came to a stop in position and exited the drivers door to open the doors for the family when to my surprise all the doors were open on my car, the jump seats were collapsed and the vehicle was empty. I looked to the limo behind mine, and it was in the same condition with me and the other driver standing in the driveway alone, the last of the family scurrying in the front door of the home. We both began to laugh because the family did all this to avoid tipping either of us. One of the wealthiest families I ever drove for gypped both drivers out of a couple dollar tip, tells me a lot about wealthy people.

I was sent to another town to pick up a body who was supposed to have been autopsied. I arrived with the removal station wagon to pick up the body and arrived at the same time as the coroner. It seemed that a prominent lawyer had been visiting a client in his suburban home when he was stricken with a cardiac arrest and died. The family reported that there was no known issues of any kind so they were anxious to learn why the father had died so suddenly. In this case I had the opportunity to be there when the autopsy was being performed. The coroner opened the chest looking for signs of heart disease by removing the heart from the chest. He needed to look no further, because when he began to slice into it on his cutting board, he saw evidence of several prior heart attacks. The heart muscle was filled with large sections of grey scar tissue surrounded by red viable tissue. The lawyer had experienced two large heart attacks before the one that killed him. The coroner sliced through his coronary arteries and found them clogged shut which was the cause of his demise. I was told to wait at the location until I could take possession of the body, so I did. Eventually, I removed the body to the funeral home, and two days later drove the family during he funeral. The wife was talking to the rabbi in the car, and she said that her husband was the picture of health, the only problem he ever had was a couple bouts of indigestion but it was several years ago. Guess what the indigestion was???

It made me squeamish

Embalming is a procedure that not many people can say they have seen. It made me squeamish at first. but after a few cases watching the embalmer is interesting. Funeral directors usually do not touch a bady themselves, they hire people to come into their place to process the bodies. The first person is usually the embalmer who brings his own tools and sometimes if the embalming fluid is not provided they bring that too. He begins by making aa cut in the side of the neck near the collar bone. He searches for the external carotid blood vessel which are pretty big and easy to locate below the skin level. Once he finds the pair, he places a stick or piece of metal like pincers under the vessels. He takes a pair of pointy scissors and snips the vessels one half way through. Into one, he places a plastic tube of the same size as the vessel, and into the other he places a large pair of 45 degree curved forceps. He then connects the tube to the preservative pump which is filled with a pink embalming fluid. He turns on the pump, and the fluid begins flowing into the body turning it pink in color every place the embalming fluid pumps into. Old clotted blood pours out of the vessel with the forceps holding it open. The pressure on the system keeps forcing the clotted blood out until it is all gone, and only embalming fluid comes out. He then removed all the neck connections and sews the neck shut. He then uses a piece of equipment called a trocar which is a round brass tube with a sword like solid point for stabbing. The shaft is filled with holes, and the handle has a hollow tube through it connecting the brass tube to the embalming fluid pump. The pump works on suction or pump and can be set to waste everything sucked out of a body which goes down a drain. The trocar is inserted into the belly button and moved in and out of the body to puncture the intestines, stomach, heart, lungs, and every other structure found in the viscera. Once everything is punctured numerous times, the suction is turned on and any fluid contains in the body cavity is sucked out and dumped. The pump is then reversed and the embalming fluid is squirted into the body cavity by the holes in the sides of the trocar tube. The tube is then removed and a small button like screw is screwed into the small hole. Attention is then turned to the mouth where a long needle is passed through the jaw below the teeth inside the mouth at the gum line. The needle is then pushed through the gums in the front of the mouth of the upper jaw. The two pieces of twine are then united by a slip know and the mouth is irrevocably sewn shut with a knot pushed inside the mouth or cheek, nothing is visible from the outside. The lips are parted and a powder is dumped into the mouth which will solidify any liquid bubbles that may try to exit the mouth. The lips are then closed tight and the body is dressed. Dressing is done the same as when you are alive for the lower half. When it comes to the shirt and coat, they are cut up the back and tucked under the body in the coffin to give the appearance that they are intact. A beautician will do both the man and the woman using make-up for each. Women have their hair done with a hot curling iron to fix just the front of the hair surrounding the face, the pillow hides the rest. The pant legs are stuffed with a v shaped cardboard giving the impression of a stand up crease in the pants leg. The body is now ready for viewing. The coffin is stuffed with usually a hay type organic material that will soak up any fluids that may leak from the body during viewing, and it will not emit any odors of any kind. Coffins are not air or water tight, and have simple latches like those on a modern window. They will not open from the inside in case you were wondering.

CRACK UP

It's a stressful line of work

The emotional and psychological strain of nursing takes a toll on the staff. Nurses cope in various ways. Some eat to relieve stress, others use drugs or alcohol, and some develop a black sense of humor. A few nurses I knew took up kickboxing as a stress reliever and one nurse engaged in target shooting. Many who cannot cope leave the field altogether. I have nurses who left nursing to become librarians, taxi cab drivers, bar tenders, real estate agents, pharmaceutical representatives, one who became a travel guide, another became mortgage broker, a sales lady in a bookstore, a cable T.V. installer and one who became a fruit picker.

I also know four nurses who had emotional breakdowns at work. One nurse was a thirty year veteran. She worked in I.C.U. and the emergency room. Eventually she was made the nurse manager of a medical-surgical floor. One day while at work she started to cry and could not stop. She ended up spending a few days in the psych unit, as a patient. Because she was a long time employee the hospital gave her a job where she reviewed charts. This is a job she seems to be handling. It involves no patient care or managerial responsibilities.

Another nurse I knew had a similar breakdown after working only five years. She spent her first year as a nurse working on a telemetry unit, then transferred to I.C.U. After working three years in I.C.U., she transferred back to telemetry because I.C.U. was becoming to stressful. Within a year of transferring back to telemetry she had a breakdown and left nursing. She froze outside of a patient's room. Eventually she went to the charge nurse and told her that she could not carry out her assignment. She left the hospital and was never seen again. The remaining nurses divided up her assignment.

Still another nurse I know recently had a breakdown, but she managed to recover and completed her shift. Half way through her assignment, that consisted of taking care of three train wrecks (a train wreck is a patient with multiple issues) she started to cry. The nurse managed to regain self control and complete the shift. She called in the next day and informed the charge nurse that she was taking a mental health day. She has returned to work.

The fourth nurse I knew that cracked up at work was a home health care coordinator. I discharge planner makes sure that the patient has all the recourses to safely recover at home. That home nursing, physical therapy and equipment (walker, hospital bed and a wound vac). This involves working with home health care agencies, insurance companies, pharmacies and durable medical equipment companies. There is also pressure by the hospital to get patients discharged in a timely manor. Eventually the stress of the job got to her and every night she came home crying. Finally her husband put his foot down and forced her to quit. After a short break, she returned to nursing reviewing charts part-time.

I have forty-three months to go before I am retired. My goal is to keep my sanity and health until retirement. I am taking it one day at a time. I tell myself all I have to do is last twelve hours. In order to keep from cracking up I sing at work. So far, I have not had any complaints from the patients. My advice to anyone going into hospital nursing is to develop a coping mechanism.